Managing Patient Flow
in Hospitals

Strategies and Solutions

Second Edition

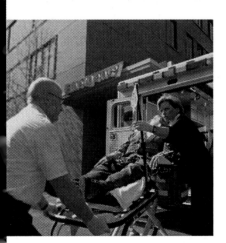 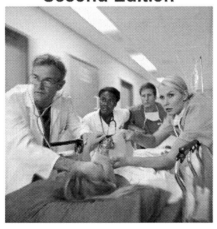 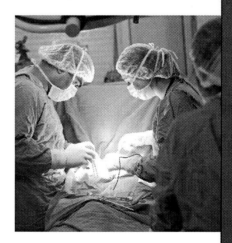

Edited by **Eugene Litvak**, Ph.D.

Foreword by **Susan Dentzer**

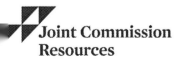
Joint Commission Resources

Executive Editor: Steven Berman

Project Manager: Christine Wyllie, M.A.

Associate Director, Production: Johanna Harris

Executive Director: Catherine Chopp Hinckley, Ph.D.

Joint Commission/JCR Reviewers: Roberta Fruth, Catherine Chopp Hinckley, Matthew Lambert, Jerod M. Loeb, Rick Morrow, Deborah M. Nadzam, Stephen Schmaltz, Paul M. Schyve, Scott Williams

Joint Commission Resources Mission

The mission of Joint Commission Resources (JCR) is to continuously improve the safety and quality of health care in the United States and in the international community through the provision of education, publications, consultation, and evaluation services.

Joint Commission Resources educational programs and publications support, but are separate from, the accreditation activities of The Joint Commission. Attendees at Joint Commission Resources educational programs and purchasers of Joint Commission Resources publications receive no special consideration or treatment in, or confidential information about, the accreditation process.

The inclusion of an organization name, product, or service in a Joint Commission Resources publication should not be construed as an endorsement of such organization, product, or service, nor is failure to include an organization name, product, or service to be construed as disapproval.

ISBN: 978-1-59940-372-4

Library of Congress Control Number: 2009932491

For more information about Joint Commission Resources, please visit http://www.jcrinc.com.

Table of Contents

I. Tutorials

II. Case Studies

Contributors

I. Tutorials

Chapter 1. The Problem of Patient Flow
Marilyn E. Rudolph, R.N., B.S.N., M.B.A., is Vice President, Performance Improvement, VHA Pennsylvania, Pittsburgh.

Chapter 2. Impact of Patient Flow Issues on Nursing Staff and Patients
Peter I. Buerhaus, Ph.D., R.N., F.A.A.N., is Valere Potter Professor of Nursing; and Director, Center for Interdisciplinary Health Workforce Studies, Institute for Medicine and Public Health, Vanderbilt University Medical Center, Nashville, Tennessee. **Anne Miller, Ph.D., R.N.,** is Assistant Professor, Center for Interdisciplinary Workforce Studies, School of Nursing, and Center for Perioperative Research in Quality, Vanderbilt University Medical Center.

Chapter 3. Assessment of Patient Flow
Brad Prenney, M.S., M.P.A., formerly Deputy Director, Program for Management of Variability in Health Care Delivery, Health Policy Institute, Boston University, Boston, is Chief Operating Officer, Institute for Healthcare Optimization, Boston.

Chapter 4. Strategies to Manage Patient Flow
Sandeep Green Vaswani, M.B.A., formerly Operations Management Consultant, Program for Management of Variability in Health Care Delivery, Health Policy Institute, Boston University, Boston, is Senior Vice President, Institute for Healthcare Optimization, Boston. **Michael C. Long, M.D.,** formerly Clinical Consultant, Program for Management of Variability in Health Care Delivery, is Senior Fellow and Clinical Consultant, Institute for Healthcare Optimization. **Brad Prenney, M.S., M.P.A.,** formerly Deputy Director, Program for Management of Variability in Health Care Delivery, is Chief Operating Officer, Institute for Healthcare Optimization. **Eugene Litvak, Ph.D.,** formerly Professor of Health Care and Operations Management and Director, Program for Management of Variability in Health Care Delivery, Boston University, is President and Chief Executive Officer, Institute for Healthcare Optimization.

Chapter 5. Measurement and Evaluation of Patient Flow: The Right Data, Measures, and Analyses
Kathleen Kerwin Fuda, Ph.D., formerly Data Analysis Manager, Program for Management of Variability in Health Care Delivery, is Senior Associate, Domestic Health Division, Abt Associates, Cambridge, Massachusetts.

II. Case Studies

Chapter 6. Cincinnati Children's Hospital Medical Center: Redesigning Perioperative Flow Using Operations Management Tools to Improve Access and Safety
Frederick C. Ryckman, M.D., is Professor of Surgery/Transplantation and Vice President of System Capacity and Perioperative Operations, Cincinnati Children's Hospital Medical Center, Cincinnati; **Elena Adler, M.D.,** is Adjunct Associate Professor, Department of Anesthesia; **Amy M. Anneken, M.S.,** is Lead Decision Support Analyst, Division of Health Policy and Clinical Effectiveness; **Cindi A. Bedinghaus,**

R.N., M.S.N., is Senior Clinical Director, Perioperative Administration; **Peter J. Clayton, M.P.A.,** is Vice President of Operations, Department of Surgical Services; **Kathryn R. Hays, M.S.N., R.N.,** is Senior Clinical Director, Perioperative Administration; **Brenda Lee, B.S.I.E.,** is Quality Improvement Manager, Division of Health Policy and Clinical Effectiveness; **Jacquelyn W. Morillo-Delerme, M.D.,** is Associate Professor, Department of Anesthesia; **Pamela J. Schoettker, M.S.,** is Medical Writer, Division of Health Policy and Clinical Effectiveness; **Paul A. Yelton** is Application Specialist III, Operating Room; and **Uma R. Kotagal, M.B.B.S., M.Sc.,** is Senior Vice President for Quality and Transformation and Director, Division of Health Policy and Clinical Effectiveness.

Chapter 7. Kaiser Permanente Southern California, Kaiser Foundation Hospital in Anaheim: Optimizing Patient Flow

Judith Kibler, R.N., M.Ed., is Senior Consultant and Lead Improvement Advisor, Kaiser Permanente (KP) Orange County, Irvine, California; and **Marlean Free, Ph.D.,** is Executive Consultant and Improvement Advisor. **Maria Lee, Ph.D., M.B.A.,** is Director of Healthcare Performance Improvement, KP Southern California, Pasadena, California; and **Kirk Rinella, M.B.A., R.C.P.,** is Program Manager, Strategic Work Environment. **Judy White** is Medical Group Administrator, KP Orange County, Anaheim and Irvine, California; and **Ed Ellison, M.D.,** is Area Medical Director. **Julie Miller-Phipps** is Executive Director and Senior Vice President, KP Hospital Health Plan, KP Orange County, Anaheim and Irvine. **Lisa Schilling, R.N., M.P.H.,** is National Vice President of Healthcare Performance Improvement and Execution Strategy, KP, Oakland, California; and a member of *The Joint Commission Journal on Quality and Patient Safety*'s Editorial Advisory Board.

Chapter 8. Northwest Community Hospital: Improving Hospitalwide Patient Flow

Barbara Weintraub, R.N., M.S.N., M.P.H., A.P.N., C.E.N., is Director, Pediatric and Adult Emergency and Trauma Services, Northwest Community Hospital, Arlington Heights, Illinois. **Kirk Jensen, M.D., M.B.A., F.A.C.E.P.,** is Chief Medical Officer, BestPractices, Inc., Fairfax, Virginia, and Faculty Member, Institute for Healthcare Improvement, Cambridge, Massachusetts. **Karen Colby, R.N., M.S., C.N.A.A.-B.C.,** is Clinical Director, Medical Pulmonary/Renal/Telemetry/Oncology Units, Northwest Community Hospital.

Foreword

Susan Dentzer

Looking back from our collective perch in the 21st century, it's clear that health care in the United States has evolved along two oddly distinct branches. Along one of them, sophisticated *clinical science* resulted in continual advances in knowledge—even if it was not always followed up by rigorous study to determine which interventions were best for patients. Along the other branch, health care has been delivered virtually without benefit of *operations management science*—which helps explain why the value of care falls short, given the trillions of dollars spent. Granted, patients aren't widgets, but as they flow through a hospital in particular, certain patterns can be identified, much as in other production systems. Yet although the science of industrial operations dates at least from the late 1800s, the notion that health care could somehow benefit from the same analyses has lagged more than a century behind.

A watershed marking a shift in this sorry state of affairs came in 2004, when The Joint Commission issued its Leadership standard for managing patient flow, Standard LD.04.03.11. The standard charged "leaders" in health care—hospital chief executive officers, trustees, and top administrative officials—with "develop[ing] and implement[ing] plans to identify and mitigate impediments to efficient patient flow throughout the hospital."* The reason for

the new standard was evident in the emerging literature: When patients aren't "flowing" well through hospitals, the result is overcrowded emergency departments, ambulance diversions, and patients being "boarded" in hallways. There's been an underlying suspicion that these developments have probably worsened patient outcomes. Yet strangely enough for a sector known for clinical science, there has been no real systematic effort to find out if that were so.

This second edition of *Managing Patient Flow in Hospitals: Strategies and Solutions*, edited by Eugene Litvak, Ph.D., highlights why health care leaders must take the issue of patient flow seriously and use proven interventions for managing it. For most hospitals, the 2007–2009 credit crunch and the accompanying recession have at least for now eliminated the option of addressing overcrowding by simply adding beds or other system capacity. (If national health care reform succeeds in slowing the flow of dollars into the health care system, that option may remain off the table for years to come.) This book, through a combination of literature

---

* The Joint Commission: *2009 Comprehensive Accreditation Manual for Hospitals: The Official Handbook.* Oakbrook Terrace, IL: Joint Commission Resources, 2008.

syntheses, tools and methods, illustrative vignettes, and real-life case studies involving particular hospitals and health systems, clearly explains why leaders must move to better-managed patient flow systems and provides a roadmap for getting there.

Opening chapters by Marilyn Rudolph (Chapter 1) and by Peter Buerhaus and Anne Miller (Chapter 2) set the stage by describing the extent of the problem of patient flow and its impact on staff and patients. Rudolph describes the consequences of suboptimal management of patient flow—that is, patients not being directed in a timely way to the best place in the hospital to care for them. It is self-evident that a patient arriving at the emergency department (ED) with a heart attack who cannot get to a cardiac catheterization laboratory fast enough may face serious danger. Yet even ED patients with less acutely emergent needs who need to be admitted may end up being boarded in a hallway or a postanesthesia care unit simply because an inpatient bed is not available. Many such patients are eventually "internally diverted" or "misplaced"—that is, assigned to a unit or bed where the level of care provided isn't optimal and "where potential safety issues, such as medical errors," as Rudolph writes, may occur. As the overload grows, elective surgeries may need to be cancelled because staff can't keep up. Those patients, needless to say, are frustrated; rescheduling open-heart surgery, after all, isn't like rescheduling a haircut. At some point, the system may become so bottlenecked that the local emergency medical system is notified that the hospital's ED will go on "ambulance diversion," meaning that any incoming emergency patients will be taken to other hospitals instead. Besides being potentially dangerous for patients, these diversions often translate into lost revenue for hospitals.

Peter Buerhaus, a leading expert on the role of nursing in health care, and his colleague Anne Miller, take the story from there. In a fictional but frighteningly realistic vignette, they show how Helen, Mark, and Sue—a nursing supervisor, unit manager, and staff nurse in a community hospital—might respond to planned and unplanned changes in patient flow in the course of a single day. Among the obstacles hurled in their path: surgeons who want to do as many surgeries as possible on Thursdays (presumably because of its proximity to the weekend); other nurses calling in sick; and a sudden influx of victims of motor vehicle accidents due to rainy weather. A "musical chairs" version of patient flow ensues—without the music, and with beds instead of chairs. Nursing overtime hours mount; and Buerhaus and Miller cite studies to remind us of links between heavy nursing hours and poor care. "Given all the events of this day," Buerhaus and Miller conclude, "it is not unreasonable to suspect that some patients were at increased risk for an adverse outcome" during their hospital stays. To add insult to injury, they add, the nursing shortage, the aging of the nursing workforce, and the declining physical abilities of older nurses make matters worse.

How to *solve* the problem of patient flow? As Brad Prenney explains in Chapter 3, the starting point is to undertake a "patient flow assessment" that analyzes "patient demand variability," the underlying cause of the systemic patient flow problems in hospitals. An assessment can enable the hospital to figure out what, if any, aspects of patient demand could be better managed to bring it in line with hospital capacity (that is, personnel, beds). For example, in the maternity ward, women who are giving birth naturally may arrive at the hospital in random patterns, while women being induced or giving birth by cesarean section could be scheduled at specific, manageable times.

Patient flow assessments are not for the data averse. Only by carefully collecting high-quality data will a hospital be able to identify the root causes of suboptimal patient flow—and trump various staff opinions that the problem is the fault of a particular unit, such as the ED. Hospitals need to analyze all sorts of data: admissions and how patients arrive—that is, through the ED, elective admissions, and transfers—what happens while patients are in the hospital (for example, are they boarded in hallways or smoothly transferred to inpatient beds?), and what care consequences ensue. The findings may be numerous and diverse, or they may not. Rest assured that they will "identify questions and issues that require further exploration," as Prenney states. But don't rest too much, because any bottlenecks identified are likely to change over time, so that patient flow assessments will have to be redone periodically.

In Chapter 4, Sandeep Green Vaswani teams with Michael Long, Brad Prenney, and Eugene Litvak to show how hospitals can use operations management science to address the patient flow issues now identified in the assessment. They drill down on the concept of variability in patient flow—especially "artificial" variability resulting from issues such as provider scheduling (get those elective surgeries done before the weekend). In fact, they identify "dysfunctional scheduling of elective admissions to a hospital" as the most significant form of artificial variability in patient "demand." As Litvak has noted, this is counterintuitive. Most ED administrators can give fairly accurate estimates of how many victims of heart attacks and gunshot wounds to plan for on a Wednesday three weeks from now, whereas a surgery administrator, when asked to estimate the number of elective surgery patients for the same day, is likely to have no clue. "Mother Nature," as he puts it, turns out to be "more predictable than our own actions."[†] It's no wonder that ED patients can't get hospital

---

† Dentzer S: Restructuring the ER, *The NewsHour with Jim Lehrer* on PBS, Jun. 7, 2005. Transcript at http://www.pbs.org/newshour/bb/health/jan-june05/er_6-07.html (accessed Sep. 8, 2009).

beds in a timely fashion on the days when the elective-surgery patients get first crack at them.

According to Vaswani et al., there's only one way to deal with this artificial variability: Eliminate it altogether. In Boston University's Program for the Management of Variability in Healthcare Delivery's three-phase approach to redesigning patient flow management, hospitals must first divide up patients into homogeneous groups (here are the elective surgery patients, here are the unscheduled admissions that come in through the ED, and so forth). Then, they must adopt new elective-surgery schedules that smooth out the flow of patients rather than bunch them up on particular days (for example, Thursdays). Finally, they must accurately estimate the resource needs, in terms of beds and staff, that will be called for at various times on various days. Critical to the entire process are "leadership commitment" from the hospital board of trustees on down and ample investment in project management expertise and data analysis.

If a patient flow management strategy is to be "science based and data driven," as Vaswani and colleagues insist, then Kathleen Kerwin Fuda, in Chapter 5, provides the tools, examples, and general advice regarding what data to collect and how to analyze them. These data form the essential foundation for a hospital's assessment of the current state of patient flow and for its identification and implementation of solutions.

Chapters 6–8 provide case studies of hospitals that have conducted patient flow assessments and then addressed the problems to improve patient flow management. In Chapter 6, a transplant surgeon, Frederick C. Ryckman, and his colleagues at Cincinnati Children's Hospital Medical Center recount patient flow problems at Children's. These problems manifested themselves in care delays and placement of children in suboptimal beds, frustrating families and clinicians. In 2006, Children's tackled patient flow to improve patient safety and increase the efficiency and reliability of care.

Using the methods described in Chapter 4, Children's began by collecting baseline data about patients being admitted. (At the time, there was no automated information system, and data were collected by hand.) Data analysis unearthed a key finding: Elective-surgical cases at Cincinnati occupied 20%–30% of the pediatric ICU beds, constituting a "significant and extremely variable portion of daily admissions and discharges."

The smoothing-out process began—again, according to the recipe, by identifying groups of similarly situated patients. Specific operating rooms were set aside each day for urgent and emergency cases, and a dedicated surgeon was appointed during these times

to handle them. The scheduling of elective surgeries was revised. Surgeons worried that the changes would cost them patients and revenues, or that the new "block" times would get in the way of their office hours or academic commitments. However, the actual outcomes were almost universally positive. Because *more* elective surgeries were done, not fewer, revenues from 2006 to June 2008 increased by 34%. Waiting times for patients decreased sharply; so did overtime hours for nurses. And, mirabile dictu, there was a "culture change in the surgical provider environment, improving mutual accountability, open communication, and team mentality."

Chapter 7 describes how Kaiser Permanente's hospital in Anaheim, California, turbocharged its efforts to improve patient flow from 2008 on. January 2008 marked a recent low point at the institution; the hospital's ED was on diversion for 302 hours, patients were boarded in the ED for 55 hours, and 1.8% of patients who came to the ED were so fed up with the wait that they went LWBS (that is, left without being seen). A widely held belief among staff was that backups in getting patients admitted to the ICU was the source of the institution's problem. Once again, a thorough data analysis pointed to different culprits, including the time it took to transfer a patient from the ICU to a bed on a medical/surgical unit. Shockingly, it seems, one unintended consequence of a move to electronic health records was that it could take as long as 20 hours for an ICU nurse to become aware that a physician had ordered a patient to be transferred out of the ICU.

A series of interventions, devised by a broad-based team that included frontline workers, succeeded in markedly cutting the average transfer time and sharply reducing variation in patient flow. Meanwhile, in a related effort, the hospital tackled another problem: speeding up patient discharges from the medical/surgical floor. A key intervention here turned out to be largely a matter of common sense. As soon as patients were admitted, nurses started asking them if they had alternate options for getting a ride home on the expected day of discharge. Partly as a result, average discharge time decreased by 26% from the first quarter of 2008 to the comparable period in 2009. (Aficionados of Southern California traffic will not be surprised to learn that transportation delays remain the most frequent cause for discharge delays from the hospital.)

Chapter 8 describes the patient flow experience at Northwest Community Hospital in Chicago's northwestern suburbs. The hospital had long struggled with patient flow problems and attempted various approaches for dealing with them, to little avail In 2007, a new emergency department medical director— evidently one named Mike, and with a good sense of humor— drew up a chart showing the tortuous, unorganized, and uninformed-by-data process that ED personnel had to undergo to locate a bed in the hospital for an ED patient. (The chart was soon named "Mike's 'Dancing with the Bed Czars.'") Patients, it seemed, had to be "pushed" through the hospital as staff tried "to coordinate a complex series of events on a schedule impossible to meet." The hospital concluded that, instead, patients should be "pulled" through the hospital, with the institution functioning as an overall system rather than as a series of discrete, and frequently warring, units.

For all the fancy theory of operations management science, the approach Northwest used was decidedly low tech. A standardized form was developed for ED personnel to request a bed. A fax line was installed so these forms could be faxed to the office of a "capacity coordinator." The hospital had no electronic bed board, so bed availability was tracked on a spreadsheet that could be viewed throughout the day on a shared computer drive. A new task force and special color-coded system was developed to provide hospitalwide alerts about looming peaks in demand. Data-driven patient flow assessments yielded valuable information on wait times, including a wide variation in when surgeries that were supposed to start at 7:30 in the morning actually got under way.

After undertaking a series of interventions, Northwest succeeded in achieving some goals and—importantly—sometimes just keeping things from getting a whole lot worse as patient census rose. Readers should come away with a fuller understanding that flow is a complex technical problem that can be far better managed than it typically is—starting, of course, with the basic approach of finding out what really is happening in the hospital.

As I write this Foreword in September 2009, it is difficult to discern the bigger picture of health reform legislation and how it may reshape health care in the United States. What is self-evident, however, is that whatever the nature and course of health reform, changes in health care delivery—within and across hospitals and other health care organizations—will be constant and ongoing. Most of those changes will take place well outside the legislative arena. Happily enough, as this book makes clear, making individual hospitals safer and far less frustrating places for patients, better places to work, and vastly more efficient users of the nation's health resources are all within our grasp.

Susan Dentzer
Editor-in-Chief, *Health Affairs*, and Health Policy Analyst, *The NewsHour with Jim Lehrer*, PBS TV

Introduction

Eugene Litvak, Ph.D.

Emergence of Patient Flow Management

If 10 years ago or so you had searched for "patient flow" on the Web, you would probably have received 100 or so URLs. Today this number exceeds 300,000. The burgeoning growth in interest in patient flow, as also seen in the emergence of a large literature, reflects widespread recognition that it is a critically important aspect of the health care delivery system in the United States and indeed throughout the world. The reasons for this interest are well known—crowded emergency departments (EDs) and excessive patient waiting times there and elsewhere, limited access to care, heavy workloads for nurses and other staff, scarce health care workforce resources, and skyrocketing health care costs. The importance of patient flow cannot be overestimated, especially in light of the current push for health care reform in the United States, because only by addressing patient flow issues can we simultaneously improve the quality and reduce the cost of health care.

The Institute for Healthcare Improvement has played a pioneering role in promoting and disseminating innovations in patient flow management.[1] The U.S. General Accountability Office, the investigative arm of the U.S. Congress, gave a strong boost to recognition of the importance of the patient flow concept in two reports, the first issued in 2003[2] and the second in 2009.[3] The more recent report indicates, for example, that the average wait time to see a physician for emergent patients was 37 minutes, more than twice as long as recommended, and that a lack of access to inpatient beds reflects competition between hospital admissions from the ED and scheduled admissions for elective surgeries. Yet it is The Joint Commission's accreditation standards that are likely the most important factor in the emergence of patient flow as an urgent concern in the health care industry. The Joint Commission's Leadership standard for managing patient flow (now Standard LD.04.03.11[4]) issued in 2004, called on hospital leaders to "develop and implement plans to identify and mitigate impediments to efficient patient flow"[5(p. 14)] throughout the hospital. Elements of performance for the Leadership standard specify, for example, that the hospital has processes that support the flow of patients throughout the hospital and uses measures of specified components of the patient flow process to assess and improve patient flow management.[4]

Purpose of This Book

This book, *Managing Patient Flow in Hospitals: Strategies and*

Solutions, second edition, is a complete revision of its predecessor, *Managing Patient Flow: Strategies and Solutions for Addressing Hospital Overcrowding*.[6] Building on the growth of theory and practice in the intervening five years, this new book provides hospitals with scientifically grounded methods to optimally manage patient flow.

Overview of Content

This book, as described by Susan Dentzer in the *Foreword*, provides a combination of literature syntheses, tools and methods, illustrative vignettes, and real-life case studies. Two of the five tutorials—Chapters 1 and 2—describe the problem of patient flow and the impact of patient flow issues on staff and patients.

The assessment and improvement strategies presented in Chapters 3 and 4 provide detailed guides on how to conduct a comprehensive assessment of patient flow and on how to use the results to identify strategies to better manage patient flow. These strategies are based on variability methodology (VM), a nonproprietary methodology developed and field tested by the authors. As Vaswani et al. state in Chapter 4, "Eliminating variability where you can and optimally managing it when you can't eliminate it is the fundamental starting point of optimally managing patient flow."[(p. 60)] Chapter 5 provides an inventory of "the right data, measures, and analyses" on which to base measurement and improvement. Accuracy of operational data is as critical to patient flow management as is accuracy of clinical data to patient care management. The readers will find some overlap among the chapters, particularly Chapters 3–5, which reflects the interrelated nature of the issues and methods at hand and the fact that most of the content represents the authors' collaborative work at the Boston University Program for Management of Variability in Health Care Delivery (MVP). This work is being further developed by four of these five authors at the newly created Institute for Healthcare Optimization (*see* http://www.ihoptimize.org). Chapter 4 provides a scientific yet very practical step-by-step guide to re-engineering patient flow. As noted in the chapter, implementing the recommendations is predicated on a hospital's resources for operations data analysis, clinical expertise, and organizational change management. Attempts to "make things easier" by not sufficiently addressing one of these components are to be discouraged—for example, as in designating an operating room for unscheduled surgeries without ensuring the availability of surgeons.

Finally, Chapters 6–8 provide detailed case studies that illustrate how three hospitals have used the measures and strategies depicted in Chapters 3–5 to successfully improve patient flow.

Who Should Read This Book?

This book will help anyone who leads or is otherwise involved in his or her hospital's efforts to improve efficiency and the flow of patients, such as the chief executive officer, chief operating officer, chief medical officer, and chief financial officer; as well as medical officers, nursing leaders, board members; medical officers; physicians, nurses, and other clinicians; quality, process improvement, and productivity managers; emergency department, surgery, critical care, and inpatient unit managers; and medical directors. Yet although this book draws on theory and practice as applied to hospitals, the patient flow management methods and tools could also be adapted to ambulatory care organizations and any other nonhospital setting. After all, all health care organizations face the challenge of balancing capacity and demand at every step in the care delivery process.

Reflections

Is reading this book *sufficient* to manage patient flow in a hospital? The answer is no. Nor would a single book enable one to become a mathematician. Is this book *necessary* for you to read if your area of expertise is patient flow—or, say, emergency nursing, finance, or quality of care—or if you are a busy health care executive or unit manager? Absolutely! Applying the patient flow management methods and tools described in this book can help to ensure that patients receive timely, high-quality care; to streamline busy EDs or ICUs; to improve nursing workloads; and to safeguard the organization's overall financial "health." These methods and tools can address patient flow problems across a wide range of settings, such as for-profit and not-for-profit hospitals and academic and community hospitals. Yet this is not a "one-size-fits-all" book. Before applying the specified strategies and solutions, conduct a comprehensive assessment to determine the unique nature of the patient flow problems at your own organization. Nor should you adopt solutions without careful consideration. For example, if you were the operating room (OR) manager or chief of surgery in a single-OR, 50-bed hospital, you would not want to reengineer your OR. Your main objective would be to investigate the source of your elective admissions, smooth these admissions, and then calculate the number of beds needed for your unscheduled medical admissions—as opposed to, say, the approach pursued by a large hospital such as Cincinnati Children's Hospital Medical Center (Chapter 6).

The issues discussed in this book are particularly important today as we grapple with the dilemma of how to improve access to care while simultaneously reducing health care costs. Unless we give up one of these goals, the only solution is to improve the efficiency of the health care delivery system so that it can serve more people with existing resources. Because efficiency depends in part on efficient management of patient flow, this book should contribute to solving the health care dilemma.

Acknowledgments

I am grateful to the co-authors of the tutorials—Marilyn E. Rudolph, R.N., B.S.N., M.B.A.; Peter I. Buerhaus, Ph.D., R.N., F.A.A.N.; Anne Miller, Ph.D., R.N.; Brad Prenney, M.S., M.P.A.; Sandeep Green Vaswani, M.B.A.; Michael C. Long, M.D.; and Kathleen Kerwin Fuda, Ph.D.—for their invaluable contributions and their patience and good humor. I would like to express my heartfelt appreciation to the enthusiastic leaders and frontline staff at Cincinnati Children's Hospital Medical Center, Cincinnati; Kaiser Permanente Southern California, Kaiser Foundation Hospital in Anaheim; and Northwest Community Hospital, Arlington Heights, Illinois, who generously share their achievements and lessons learned in this book's case studies. I am also indebted to Susan Dentzer for providing her insightful and engaging Foreword. I extend my sincere gratitude to the editor, Steven Berman, whose constant attention and tireless work made the final version of the book significantly better than our first draft, and to the executive director of the Department of Publications, Catherine Chopp Hinckley, Ph.D., at Joint Commission Resources, for their guidance and support.

I am indebted to Harvey V. Fineberg, M.D., Ph.D., my former dean at the Harvard School of Public Health (currently president of the Institute of Medicine of the National Academies) for his continuing support and guidance. Without him, my career would have definitely taken a very different path, and I would not be having the pleasure of investigating patient flow. I am also very grateful to Donald M. Berwick, M.D., IHI president and chief executive officer, a colleague and advisor of many years, who recognized early on the importance of patient flow to the field of quality and patient safety and who has played a leading role in its development and implementation. Finally, I would like to thank my mother, Anna, for managing me for many years (an even more difficult task than managing patient flow); my wife, Ella, for many important things in my life that have nothing to do with this book; and my son, Mark, whose companionship constantly reminds me that the time I have not spent on patient flow can also be rewarding.

References

1. Institute for Healthcare Improvement: *Optimizing Patient Flow: Moving Patients Smoothly Through Acute Care Settings*. IHI Innovation Series white paper. Boston: Institute for Healthcare Improvement, 2003 (available on www.IHI.org; accessed Sep. 8, 2009).

2. U.S. General Accountability Office: *Hospital Emergency Departments: Crowded Conditions Vary Among Hospitals and Communities*, Mar. 2003. http://www.gao.gov/new.items/d03460.pdf (accessed Sep. 8, 2009).

3. U.S. General Accountability Office: *Hospital Emergency Departments: Crowding Continues to Occur, and Some Patients Wait Longer Than Recommended Time Frames*, Apr. 2009. http://www.gao.gov/new.items/d09347.pdf (accessed Sep. 8, 2009).

4. The Joint Commission: *2009 Comprehensive Accreditation Manual for Hospitals: The Official Handbook*. Oakbrook Terrace, IL: Joint Commission Resources, 2008.

5. The Joint Commission: New Leadership standard on managing patient flow for hospitals. *Joint Commission Perspectives* 24:13–14, Feb. 2004.

6. The Joint Commission: *Managing Patient Flow: Strategies and Solutions for Addressing Hospital Overcrowding*. Oakbrook Terrace, IL: Joint Commission Resources, 2004.

Section I. Tutorials

Chapter 1

The Problem of Patient Flow

Marilyn E. Rudolph, R.N., B.S.N., M.B.A.

Every day in hospitals, patients are admitted, discharged, and transferred from unit to unit. When patient flow is optimal, daily work proceeds throughout the hospital at a steady pace. When patient flow is suboptimal, issues arise, troops are rallied, and concerns are voiced by patients, physicians, nurses, and other caregivers, as well as administrative leaders. Inherently, inefficient patient flow has far-reaching effects on patient care and on multiple aspects of the hospital's operations, quality, patient safety, and potential revenue.

According to a recent U.S. General Accountability Office report, emergency departments (EDs) in hospitals in the United States are crowded, resulting in ambulance diversions, long wait times, and boarding (holding patients in beds or hallways after the decision to admit).[1] Until recently, the ED was held up as being the crux of patient flow problems in almost every hospital. Staff who work in the ED know this all too well: "If we fix the ED, we'll fix patient flow, right?" Wrong! For example, conversations with participants in a flow management collaborative[2] indicated that they quickly realized or confirmed that although the effects of inadequate patient flow are manifested in the ED, patient flow issues are systemwide.

To compound the problem of inefficiencies and variability in patient flow, health care systems now face strenuous economic challenges not previously experienced. The current economic distress has intensified the need to address many of the consequences when patient flow isn't adequate, let alone optimal. Inefficient patient flow and, more importantly, the consequent diminishing throughput—that is, the number of patients per unit of time—can adversely affect an organization's financial health and viability.

Leaders should be conversant with The Joint Commission Leadership standard on managing patient flow, Standard LD.04.03.11: "Leaders develop and implement plans to identify and mitigate impediments to efficient patient flow throughout the hospital."[3(pp. LD-22–LD-23)] In response, hospitals are increasingly ensuring that senior leadership and boards of directors are knowledgeable and actively engaged regarding the challenging patient flow, utilization, and capacity issues. If senior leaders and board trustees are not engaged regarding the financial, clinical, and perceptual implications associated with inefficient patient flow and throughput, the organization may be at risk for suboptimal performance in these areas. Northwest Community Hospital (Arlington Heights, IL; see Chapter 8), for example, provides data on a quarterly basis to trustees and senior leadership on a variety of patient flow–related issues and process improvements. The metrics are included on a dashboard for key goals in the hospital's overall operating plan; some of them are as follows:

- Revise bed management process, including use of automatic bed board system
- Define and establish data set of information needed to place patients in the right inpatient beds
- Review top diagnosis-related groups (DRGs) and case-mix index to identify areas of opportunity for LOS reductions, blended (average LOS goal, 3.28 days)
- Left Without Being Seen (LWBS; goal, < 1%)
- Internal and External Diversions (goal, 0)

The data for two of these metrics, as provided in the key goals dashboard, are shown in Figure 1-1 (page 5).

Until recently, it was common for hospitals to attempt to address overcrowding by adding beds to the ED and inpatient areas. Yet adding beds is no longer an option for many hospitals, given current constraints on capital spending. In addition, adding beds could even exacerbate the problem by creating more room for boarders.[4]

The gravity of the current financial situation and its impact on hospitals in terms of cuts, delays, and reviews regarding capital spending are represented in the views of chief financial officers (CFOs),[5] who, for example, have "reduced five-year capital spending by almost a third" or "deferred purchases of capital equipment, only replacing equipment that becomes inoperable." Addressing patient flow–related capacity issues will most likely continue to present a large challenge, given the overall need to maintain viable or growing revenue streams for most hospitals both in the near and the distant future. Therefore, capital spending to support organizational improvements will also likely remain an issue.

Also related to patient flow is the high cost of staffing, including the inflationary pressure on costs due to nurse shortages (which may be alleviated by the recent increase in employment [*see* Chapter 2]). Nurses may often experience the uncomfortable effects of variable census or staffing shortages, so that when there are insufficient staff to care for patients, or when the census rises, their own workloads increase. The current variability in staffing needs on a day-to-day or week-to-week basis is quite challenging to both administrators and caregivers (*see* Chapter 2), and the tendency is to default to average staffing needs to help reduce costs and then do what is needed to increase staff in times of peak census. Up-and-down staffing requirements, an undesired result of the wide variations in patient throughput, are commonly recognized, expected, and even accepted in response to the peaks and valleys of patient census.

Nurse executives, hospital managers, and other leaders who deal with the multiple problems associated with staffing needs that fluctuate daily should consider the following questions[6]:

- Are all the peaks in the demand pattern for hospital care inevitable?
- Are they all patient driven, or are they at least partly the result of uninformed or less-than-optimal management?
- Does today's economic reality mean that we cannot achieve both adequate nurse staffing and affordable cost?

As the following CFO responses[5] indicate, administrators know that hospital service lines are under increasing pressure to show measured results that reflect favorable productivity and efficiency:

- "We are making major investments to improve our own efficiency and productivity. We are combining this with investments in training and our people." (100- to 300-bed stand-alone hospital)
- "Reengineering services to reduce costs." (100- to 300-bed, stand-alone hospital)
- "Implemented a tighter productivity standard for daily monitoring." (100- to 300-bed hospital)
- "Ensure profitable service lines have the tools they need." (100- to 300-bed hospital)

The current financial situation lends urgency to the need to deliver the best possible care as cost-effectively and profitably as possible. Diversion of patients from the ED and cancellation of elective surgical procedures represent two examples of how patient flow–related issues adversely affect profitability and, potentially, the quality and safety of patient care at the service-line level. The impact of problems associated with patient flow are now examined in greater detail.

Census Peaks and Valleys

As ups and downs in patient census occur, caregivers and administrators work creatively to rally to the peaks and gear down for the valleys. The tendency in health care is to accept these frequent fluctuations, but should peaks and valleys in patient census be acceptable, considering the potential adverse impact of fluctuations, especially peaks, on patient care?

Patient throughput issues hinge on the peaks and valleys of the inpatient census. In high-demand inpatient areas (for example, critical care, telemetry, and surgical units), nurses and other caregivers bear the brunt of the spikes in patient census that can occur on a day-to-day, week-to-week, or season-to-season basis. In addition to the day-to-day and week-to-week variability, the potential exists for more than one patient to occupy a single bed (currently, not

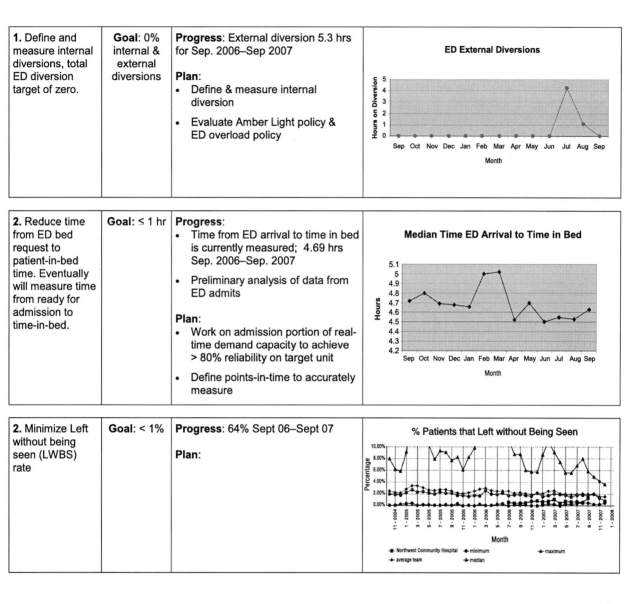

Figure 1-1. Data for Two Metrics on Dashboard, Northwest Community Hospital

Data for two metrics are shown from its key goals dashboard. ED, emergency department.

Source: *Provided courtesy of Barbara Weintraub, Director, Emergency Department, Northwest Community Hospital, Arlington Heights, Illinois. Used with permission.*

at the same time!) on any particular day, possibly adding hour-to-hour variability to patient census and nursing workload.

Unnecessary patient turnover, which occurs when a patient is placed in a bed because it was available and not necessarily because it was the optimal unit for that patient's care (*see* Sidebar 1-1, page 6), reflects system throughput inefficiencies. In turn, it generates the potential for added work and increased handoffs (handovers) for inpatient unit nurses, when one takes into

account the patient's later transfer to the optimal unit when a bed becomes available. The scenario depicted in Sidebar 1-1 is not unusual and is likely to occur daily in many hospitals, as patient census and bed demand fluctuates.

The opportunity to efficiently prioritize individual workloads may be diminished or compromised because nurses really aren't certain what their patient census might be at a given point in time throughout the workday or workweek. When nurses cannot

Sidebar 1-1. Mr. Jones and Mrs. Smith

A patient, Mr. Jones, was to have orthopedic surgery at 9 A.M. (09:00) and be admitted to the orthopedic unit after his recovery. Mr. Jones's orthopedic surgery is delayed until 11 A.M., (11:00), so the nurse assigned to that bed on the orthopedic surgical unit is sent a medical admission, Mrs. Smith, with acute heart failure. Mrs. Smith is sent to the surgical unit from the ED because there are currently no beds available on the heart failure unit, and she has been waiting in the ED for an inpatient bed since the previous evening. The nurse completes the admission interview, the paperwork, and all immediate care needs for Mrs. Smith, only to then be told that a bed is now available on the heart failure unit and that Mrs. Smith is to be transferred. The same nurse then completes the transfer activities, and Mrs. Smith leaves the unit. The orthopedic unit bed is now available for Mr. Jones, the surgical patient, and he is transferred to the open bed, and this occurs just before shift change, and the same nurse now must complete the entire admission workup for Mr. Jones! If the optimal bed had been available for Mrs. Smith when originally needed, the one orthopedic nurse's workload would have been more far more predictable and manageable.

predict patient census during the workday or over the workweek, the opportunity to efficiently prioritize individual workloads may be compromised. For example, consider the vignette described in Sidebar 1-1.

Figure 1-2 (below) reflects significant variability in one hospital's elective surgical admission population on a day-to-day basis during a four-week period. This level of daily variability presents challenges in efficient patient placement, staffing of postoperative inpatient care units, and planning for the need for other support staff and services.

The traditional approach to use the midnight patient census may misrepresent the actual daily census, activity, and workloads. The census variability throughout the day can present significant demands on staff and resources. How to best count daily patient census is an enduring question for most hospitals, but a far more appropriate question to ask is How do we best minimize patient census peaks and valleys so that workloads become far more predictable from hour to hour, day to day, week to week, and season to season?

Caregivers inherently know that eliminating significant census peaks and valleys, such as those seen in Figure 1-2, is critical to improving patient flow and resource utilization, but the question that often arises is How can this be done?

Resource Utilization

The deployment and utilization of resources such as staffing are an ongoing challenge in most organizations. Patient flow is a key driver of capability to most appropriately determine what resources—both human and physical—are needed to best serve patients. Most caregivers and nurse leaders readily acknowledge

that they struggle almost daily to identify the ideal set of resources needed to care for patients.

Variation in resource utilization directly or indirectly affects every department, staff member, patient, and budget within a hospital. Joan Massella, administrative vice president and chief nursing officer at St. Clair Hospital (Mt. Lebanon), located in western Pennsylvania, explains, "One challenge is to help all caregivers understand that patient flow and the effect on resources is a system issue and not an individual unit or department issue."[7]

With that thought in mind, it is useful to think about patient flow from the perspective of the Joint Commission's on-site tracer methodology, in which a surveyor follows the flow or route of a patient through an entire organization to assess compliance with various standards in multiple areas providing patient care.[8] Chapter 2 explains the wide impact of the variability in patient flow on the resources needed for patient care and services. Clinicians and managers are at a significant disadvantage in

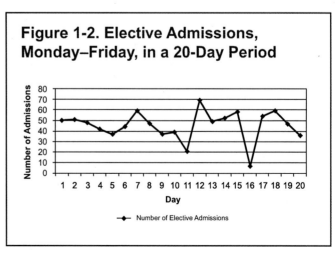

This figure shows the number of elective surgical admissions for Monday through Friday for a 20-day period.

planning for resource needs with limited control on patient flow. Patient acuity is also a factor to be considered in resource utilization. As the patient's severity of illness increases, the demand for resources also increases. Department directors, nurse leaders, administrators, and the many other persons who support, directly or indirectly, the system of patient care, are challenged to manage resources *to match to the peaks and valleys* rather than *optimally manage the peaks and valleys systemwide.* The challenge reaches beyond the single patient to system operations as the organization attempts to develop optimal delivery of services. As long as hospitals tolerate even moderately wide census peaks and valleys, the readily accepted workaround or quick fix of off-service patient placement ("internal diversion") brings its own challenges to physicians, nurses, and other staff.

Internal Diversion

Internal diversion, as illustrated in Sidebar 1-1, occurs when a patient is assigned to a patient care unit or bed that is not considered to be the optimal location in which a patient would receive the highest standards of disease-specific care for his or her diagnosis. Internal diversion, along with the associated and added transfers and handoffs, often occurs in times of high demand for a select service and/or in times of high census housewide. Caregivers, usually nurses with optimal skills to care for a select patient population, might not be available to care for these patients when they are placed in off-service settings. In the vignette in Sidebar 1-1, the nurse, a skilled and competent orthopedic nurse, found herself caring for a patient who was identified as one who would most likely be better served in the designated acute heart failure unit.

Caregivers recognize internal diversion as a potential compromise to providing the best care when specialty units such as postoperative specialty units, ICUs, and telemetry units are not used as originally intended. At times, a physician might request that a patient be sent to a preferred or select unit, such as ICU or telemetry, because of a higher level of comfort with or knowledge about the nature of care delivery in the unit. For example, patients who do not require specialized care may be placed in specialty units, or worse, patients needing specialty care may not have a bed available when needed and may therefore be placed in alternate units for the duration of their stay or until a specialty bed becomes available. When the patient is transferred to the optimal unit, another handoff occurs for the nurses, as in the vignette in Sidebar 1-1, which might compromise patient care. Patient safety concerns—and staff satisfaction to a lesser extent—should prompt a closer look at patient placement and internal diversion. As hospitals become more crowded, the price of ignoring such variability

will more clearly manifest itself in unmet patient needs and diminished quality.[9]

Many organizations designate specialty care units with the intent of providing the highest quality of patient care. Nurses and other caregivers acquire and build on the needed skills, experience, and knowledge, often attaining certification to care for patients with injuries or disease-specific conditions that are assigned to the specialty care units. Caregivers who choose to work in these areas may become dissatisfied because they feel that their specialty skills are not being fully utilized when they deliver care to off-service patients who do not require a higher level of skilled care. On the other hand, caregivers' skill sets may be stretched when not delivering care to patients in their own specialty units, such as in the vignette in Sidebar 1-1. This is when potential safety issues, such as medical errors, and failure to deliver identified standards of care may occur. Thus, internal diversion potentially has far-reaching effects on staff and on patients.

Although not all hospitals track the number of internal diversions, such data, as shown in Figure 1-3 (page 8), are worth collecting. Yet many hospitals do not collect internal diversion data because they might not recognize internal diversion as a potential compromise in patient safety or appropriate care. Hospitals usually collect such data because they are aware that internal diversion is an issue and are willing to determine how they can get the right patient in the right bed every time.

The possible secondary effects of off-service patient placement—such as patient care issues and adverse outcomes, staff and physician satisfaction, added transfers and handoffs, rework, readmissions, and medical errors—are usually not measured as they directly or indirectly relate to off-service patient placement. Administrators should consider that it may be difficult to assess the potentially negative impact of off-service patient placement across multiple areas of the organization without monitoring or measuring internal diversion. Medical errors could be monitored as a balancing measure for internal diversion. Currently, most organizations do not try to correlate their patient population that is placed in off-service units or issues with patient flow to medical errors.

Increases in Medical Errors

The potential for medical errors is certainly of concern, given that variable patient flow contributes to the stress on caregivers. According to the Institute of Medicine (IOM),[10] research shows that most medical errors are preventable and are system related. (The IOM defines *medical error* as "the failure to complete a

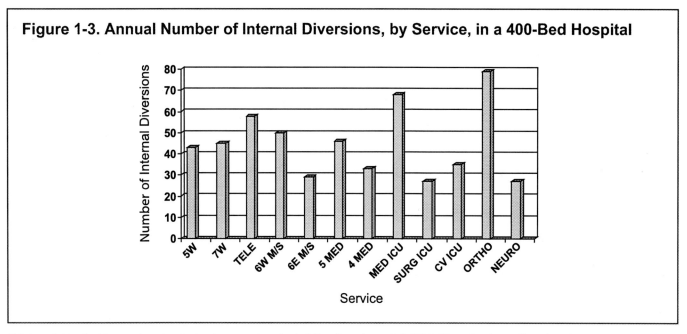

Figure 1-3. Annual Number of Internal Diversions, by Service, in a 400-Bed Hospital

This hospital tracked the number of patients who were placed or held in off-service units in 2008. The units where off-service placement occurred were as follows: 5 West, 7 West, Telemetry, 6 West medical/surgical, 6 East medical/surgical, 5 Medical, 4 Medical, Medical ICU, Surgical ICU, Cardiovascular ICU, Orthopedics, and Neurology. Used with permission.

planned action as intended or the use of a wrong plan to achieve an aim").[10 (p. 28)] The question to consider is Do the stresses of patient flow cause any caregiver to inadvertently fail to complete a planned action as intended or use a wrong plan to achieve an aim? If this question were posed to individuals directly or indirectly involved in patient care, the response from the majority most likely would be "quite possibly," with others providing a resounding "yes" response (*see* Chapter 2 for research findings). Variability in throughput, with frequent peaks in bed utilization, create system stresses, such as higher staffing demands in all areas of an organization. Yet it is most likely that the major stresses are frequently experienced by nurses and other caregivers who directly provide patient care. Burdensome workloads and staff shortages that can occur when bed utilization is repeatedly at a maximum may lead to nurses working overtime (more than 40 hours a week). The likelihood of making an error increases with longer work hours—and is three times higher when nurses work shifts lasting 12.5 hours or more. In addition, the risks of making an error increase significantly when nurses work overtime.[11]

Delays in Patient Care

Decreased or delayed throughput can be associated with delays in patient care and services rendered. Patients and their families have expectations for expedient service and readily become exasperated with even minimal waits and delays in treatment or care, and they certainly experience greater frustration as care delays are prolonged. Caregivers want to provide care that will meet the needs

of patients in a timely and efficient manner, but the variability in patient census affects their control of work flow.

Delays in care in the ED are of major concern to patients, caregivers, and managers. Events that may trigger patient care delays in the ED could be related to a very busy ED, but according to one hospital administrator, "It is crucial to understand that most of the throughput delays are due to downstream bottlenecks."[12] That is, the unavailability of inpatient beds reflects inefficient throughput processes, high inpatient-bed utilization, and/or peaks in census. One or more of these scenarios could occur at any given time, possibly resulting in delays in treatment and care for patients.

Thrombolytic or interventional therapies for stroke or acute myocardial infarction, prompt management of asthma or other respiratory ailments, antibiotic administration, and pain relief are just a few examples of treatments or care that are time sensitive and may be adversely affected by ED delays. According to David Kish, executive director of emergency services and patient logistics, St. Clair Hospital:

> Delays in service and care potentially put patients at risk. That's the bottom line. Do we always know what is going on with patients in the waiting room? Even if it isn't life threatening, delays create dissatisfied patients.[13]

It is well recognized that patients with emergent and urgent needs are prioritized and receive expedited care, but all patients who present to an ED expect prompt treatment in what they perceive to be a reasonable time frame. Care delays can affect many patients in many ways—from the ultimate delay that may result in an inadvertent patient death to a delay that causes added discomfort or anxiety for patients and their families. ED physicians and nurses are just as frustrated by delays in care as patients are and certainly want the delays to be addressed sooner rather than later and in an appropriate manner. Yet they may also have limited ability to mitigate the downstream bottlenecks that could be directly or indirectly contributing to care delays.

Boarders and ED Diversion

Delays in transferring patients to an inpatient unit from the ED, a postanesthesia care unit (PACU), an outpatient cardiac catheterization laboratory or radiology procedure, or an observation unit frequently present challenging situations to the staff and unsatisfactory experiences for the patients. If delays in moving patients into an inpatient bed are significant, patients are held in these areas as boarders. The situation of temporarily holding or boarding a patient in an area until an appropriate bed is available creates concerns for patients, families, and staff. ED diversion, when hospitals determine that their EDs can no longer accept ambulance patients for a designated amount of time because of overcrowding, is often associated with the boarding of patients. Figure 1-4 (below) demonstrates the LOS for each patient boarded in one acute care ED during a one-month time frame.

The boarding of patients can potentially lead to quality of care and safety issues, breeches in standards of care, treatment delays, privacy concerns, and errors for the patients being boarded and for the other patients also being served in crowded or suboptimal

settings. In view of the safety concerns associated with a crowded ED, some hospitals have determined that boarding patients in hallways of inpatient units is preferable to boarding patients in the ED. The rationale for this decision is that sending patients to an inpatient unit is preferred because caring for one patient in a less-than-ideal setting (a hallway) is less risky than caring for numerous boarded patients in an already overcrowded and extremely busy ED. For example, 540-bed Stony Brook University Hospital, which has instituted hallway boarding, has found that the vast majority of patients prefer to wait for a bed on the inpatient unit rather than in the ED.[14]

Boarded ED patients may increase ED nurse-to-patient staffing ratios considerably, whereas placing a single patient in a hallway for one nurse to care for on an inpatient care unit may not significantly increase the nurse-to-patient ratio. The pros and cons of boarding patients in hallways have been much debated, and organizations are making what they consider to be the best decisions as these situations arise. Yet boarders, whether in the ED or in hallways, are still a considerable source of frustration for caregivers and administrators, and they generate concerns regarding patient safety.

Another decision that comes into play when ED overcrowding and boarding occur is whether to invoke diversion status when the ED can no longer accept ambulance arrivals because of very high utilization or overcrowded conditions in the ED and/or inpatient areas. Interestingly, as Eugene Litvak and colleagues have demonstrated, boarding is likely to be more rather than less prevalent when the ED is on diversion status. In comparing the average number of boarders in the ED during nondiversion and diversion

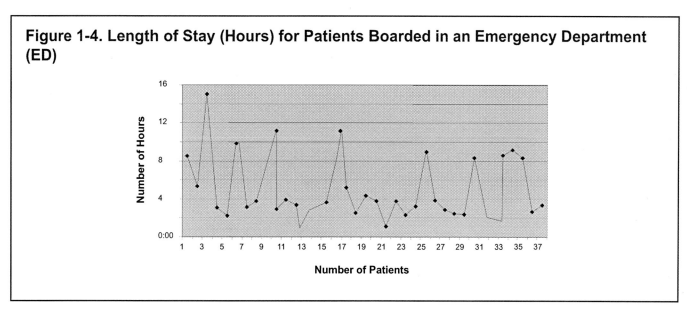

Figure 1-4. Length of Stay (Hours) for Patients Boarded in an Emergency Department (ED)

The length of stay, shown in the y axis, for 38 patients (x axis) boarded in one acute care ED during a one-month time frame is shown. Used with permission.

hours, they found that across two hospitals, EDs in nondiversion averaged 4.03 patient boarders per hour, while EDs in diversion averaged 7.16 patient boarders per hour, a 78% increase.[15] Not surprisingly, this tells us that during diversion hours, about one-third of ED bed capacity was taken up by boarded patients. Furthermore, as shown in Figure 1-5 (right), as the number of patients boarding in the ED increases, so does diversion. Litvak et al. suggest that boarders may be the most significant contributing factor to ED diversion.[15]

Nurse leaders of inpatient PACUs and surgical departments report in personal conversations an increase in boarding of postoperative surgical patients in the PACU for a few hours to overnight. Many organizations attribute PACU boarders to high surgical volumes and to the inability to transfer patients to appropriate units because inpatient beds are not available when needed. Lack of availability of critical care beds for postoperative patients creates a significant change in PACU work flow and increases the risk to boarder patients.

Patient diversions, both internal and external, as well as boarding of patients create stress in hospital systems. As in the ED, boarding patients in a PACU generates concerns related to staffing, resource consumption, added costs, and, of course, patient, staff and physician satisfaction. Rendering care to patients in a less-than-ideal setting by boarding them is not the preferred or chosen manner in which to deliver services, but boarding in PACUs, EDs, and hallways may continue to occur as long as census peaks and valleys and the causative factors of patient flow variability are tolerated and not fully addressed.

Left Without Being Seen

Patients who present to the ED expect to be seen and treated by a health care professional expeditiously. In an ED boarding situation, the majority of patients who are boarded choose to remain in the hospital and tolerate the boarding until a bed becomes available. On the other hand, waiting ED patients, not having received care in a time frame acceptable to them, may tire of further waiting for care and then leave the ED before receiving treatment. These patients are categorized as LWBS.

The quality and safety implications for LWBS can range from patient dissatisfaction and deterioration in the patients' condition to delays in care or care that is never provided to patients in need. Hospital administrators find this to be a particularly disturbing occurrence from a quality and safety perspective and also realize the possible revenue and legal implications, including possible violation of the patient anti-dumping statute.[16]

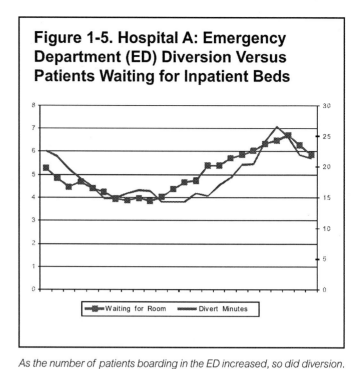

Figure 1-5. Hospital A: Emergency Department (ED) Diversion Versus Patients Waiting for Inpatient Beds

As the number of patients boarding in the ED increased, so did diversion.

Source: Litvak E., McManus M.L., Cooper A.: A Root Cause Analysis of Emergency Department Crowding and Ambulance Diversion in Massachusetts. *Boston University Program for the Management of Variability in Health Care Delivery, Report to the Massachusetts Department of Public Health, Oct. 2002. http://www.mass.gov/Eeohhs2/docs/dph/quality/healthcare/ad_emergency_dept_analysis.doc.*

Like diversion and boarding, LWBS occurrences may reflect ED overcrowding. According to one survey, 2% of patients leave the ED without being seen by a health care provider.[17] According to a U.S. General Accountability Office report (2003), LWBS ranges from 3% to 5%.[18] Figure 1-6 (page 11) shows one hospital's monthly LWBS data, representing an average of 4.3% for this hospital.

Most acute care EDs have some experience with the LWBS population. According to an ED spokesperson at one hospital, "overcrowding, long waits, and frustrated staff and patients had become commonplace." That hospital's LWBS rate was about 3%—at the low end of LWBS range compared to the example above—but still sufficient to be of concern to administrators. David Kish has said the following about the LWBS population:

> It is tempting to say, and I've heard comments such as "If they left without being seen, they couldn't have been that sick." In reality, many patients who leave without being seen are sick. Patients come to the emergency room because they feel that they have no other recourse or they aren't sure of the severity of their illness. That is why we are there as health professionals. Furthermore, from a financial standpoint, the lost revenue from LWBS patients can be significant.[13]

In addition to the quality and safety issues associated with inefficient patient flow, inefficient throughput may also compromise sources of revenue that are critical to a hospital's ability to maintain acceptable operating margins. Administrators must also give consideration to the anti-dumping statute, which may place added requirements and obligations on hospitals to address the LWBS population, thus potentially adding work to an already stressed system of care.

Decreased Throughput and Lost Revenue

Inefficiencies in patient flow are frequently a manifestation of hospitals functioning at full capacity or nearly so. Often, administrators strive for and encourage high bed occupancy and utilization in the belief that they are best for business, but this is not the reality. In actuality, as utilization increases to above a functional capacity that is safe, manageable, appropriate, efficient, and conducive to optimal throughput, system inefficiencies occur and become apparent in a detrimental manner—reduced throughput and revenue—just the opposite of what one might expect.

It is very apparent that the reason hospitals exist is to provide care to patients. However, a reality of care delivery is that patients, for the most part, generate the revenue that helps to keep hospitals solvent and functional so that the hospitals can continue to serve their communities in the best manner possible. Therefore, it is necessary to acknowledge the potentially considerable revenue losses associated with ED diversions and/or cancellations of

elective procedure cases (primarily surgical). For example, a 450-bed nonprofit community teaching hospital in York, Pennsylvania, identified a practical method for quantifying potential revenue loss as a result of LWBS occurrences and ambulance diversion. Data from 62,588 patient visits to the ED in a one-year period (July 2004–June 2005) suggested that the hospital lost $3,881,506 in net revenue as a result of ambulance diversions and LWBS occurrences.[19] In another study, 10,301 adult, nontrauma ED patients arriving by ambulance in 2002 and 2003 averaged hospital revenues of $4,492, and each hour spent by a patient on diversion was associated with $1,086 of lost revenue from ambulance patients.[20]

Just as important as revenue losses from ED diversions are the losses associated with cancelled elective surgical procedures. Cancellations in times of very high inpatient bed utilization are usually made to maintain a safe patient care environment—that is, to avoid possible compromise of care for current or future patients. Yet most organizations are very hesitant, even unwilling, to cancel scheduled procedures, given the subsequent dissatisfaction of patients and surgeons. Patients and their family members often take time off from work to accommodate the planned surgical procedure and recovery time; futhermore, patients have followed the protocol for preparing themselves for the surgery and experience the anxiety, risk, and inconvenience when the surgical procedure is cancelled. Costs are incurred by the hospital, the surgeon, and other providers, such as the anesthesiologist.

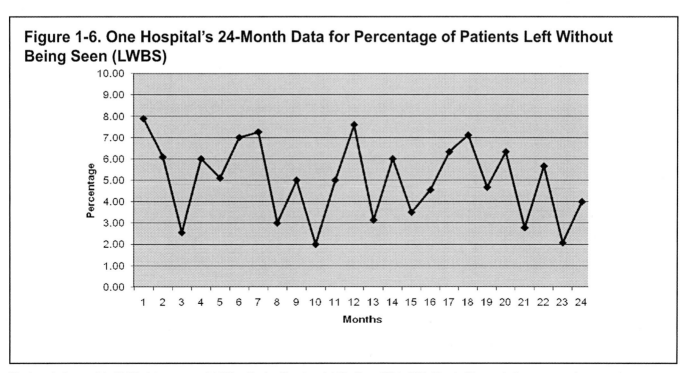

Figure 1-6. One Hospital's 24-Month Data for Percentage of Patients Left Without Being Seen (LWBS)

The hospital's monthly LWBS data averaged 4.3%, with significant variability (from 2% to 8%). Used with permission.

A recent article that reports on the experience at Launceston General Hospital in Tasmania, Australia, portrays the kind of struggle that occurs when hospital executives need to determine whether elective surgeries should be cancelled.[21] Some 19 elective surgery cases were cancelled in May and June 2009, compared with 2 or 3 during an average month. Nursing overtime, the need to board patients, and competition for beds together resulted in a "hospitalwide bed jam," which led the hospital to cancel elective surgeries as the "only bed management tool available."

Potential revenue losses for a cancelled surgical case for hospitals in the United States that are not on a fixed annual budget average $1,430 to $,1700 per OR hour; for hospitals with a fixed annual budget (for example, Department of Veterans Affairs hospitals) or hospitals outside the United States, cancelling a case and performing it on another day increases costs to the physicians, hospital, patient, and society, even if overtime would have been required to perform the case on the day it was originally scheduled.[22]

After a surgical case is cancelled, it might not be rescheduled in the same institution. In one study, 145 (11%) of the 1,294 scheduled cases in 2000 in a busy university hospital's vascular surgical service were cancelled and not performed on the original day of schedule. Sixty-six (46%) of the 145 cancellations were due to nonmedical reasons. Ninety (62%) of the 145 cancellations were rescheduled, 29 (20%) resulted in different surgeries, and the remaining 6 (4%) patients had no surgeries at the hospital. The results suggest that better scheduling might have prevented cancellations and resulted in savings of unnecessary costs.[23] In addition to decreased throughput and lost revenue, increased LOS is another consequence of less-than-optimally managed patient flow.

Increased Length of Stay

Extended LOS has always been of concern to hospitals, but the need to optimize LOS to prevent lengthy hospitalization for all patients is especially critical in the current economic situation. Turning over beds more frequently without compromising patient care maximizes revenue, so efficient patient flow—and greater throughput—is of higher priority today than ever before.

All the problems associated with patient flow discussed so far in this chapter—from census peaks and valleys through decreased throughput—can potentially contribute to extended LOS. For example, whereas the average LOS in telemetry, step-down, or monitored care units ranges from three to five days in many organizations, the LOS in the telemetry unit represented in Figure 1-7 (page 13) is considerably higher, reflecting the hospital's inability to effectively move patients in a congested, inefficiently flowing system.

Reducing LOS by 0.25 days in a typical 300-bed hospital, for example, can result in a functional increase of 12 beds.[24] In addition to the possibility of lost revenue when beds are not turned over efficiently, consideration should also be given to patient satisfaction issues associated with extended LOS. Although some patients might prefer to stay in the hospital as long as possible, most patients want to return to their preferred and familiar environments.

Staff and Patient Satisfaction

Hospital leaders agree that improving satisfaction among physicians, nurses, other staff, and patients is a key organizational strategy and that reducing delays associated with patient flow—without adversely affecting quality and financial performance—is an important area of focus. Satisfaction among nurses and other caregivers, as stated earlier, may be adversely affected by internal diversion of patients. Physicians prefer that patients be placed in appropriately designated units to receive optimal care according to identified standards.

Patient satisfaction, especially regarding quality of bedside care and on-time performance, can also reflect the problems associated with patient flow. In improving the efficiency of patient flow, St. Clair Hospital referred to patient satisfaction scores to help identify areas of particular concern. For example, a commercially available satisfaction survey showed St. Clair's ED mean patient satisfaction score for door-to-room time of 68 (versus an average of 73.8 for the peer comparison group). In addition, its ED door-to-physician time of 80 minutes was 20 minutes higher than that of the peer comparison group. By taking action on the identified opportunities for improvement in patient flow, St. Clair was able to address many of its patient flow issues. For example, ED door-to-physician time improved by 60%, door-to-room time improved by 85%, and mean patient satisfaction scores increased to 87.1 (versus a peer-group mean of 74.7).[25]

Many other hospital leaders could relate to and have spoken about these very same throughput issues and their contribution to patient dissatisfaction. As long as there are inefficiencies in patient throughput that are reflected in less-than-optimal satisfaction scores, organizational leaders will attempt to improve patient throughput in multiple areas of the acute care system.

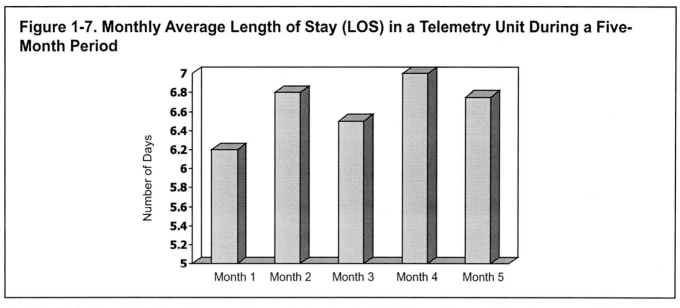

Figure 1-7. Monthly Average Length of Stay (LOS) in a Telemetry Unit During a Five-Month Period

As depicted in the figure, the LOS for a telemetry unit for a randomly selected period of five months was well above the average, which could reflect diversion of patients who would be better placed in a medical/surgical unit or a high-demand unit, such as the ICU. Used with permission.

Reflections

Clearly, suboptimal patient flow has many consequences in terms of quality and safety and in terms of financial and operational performance. Health care leaders must acknowledge that especially in today's economic environment, throughput issues, systemwide inefficiencies, and the potential consequences for patient care are compelling reasons to work toward eliminating as much variability in patient flow in health care systems as possible. Now might well be the time for them to take immediate action to optimize patient flow. The benefits to be gained in quality, safety, efficiency, and revenue are considerable, as discussed in subsequent chapters of this book.

References

1. U.S. General Accountability Office (GAO): *Hospital Emergency Departments: Crowding Continues to Occur, and Some Patients Wait Longer Than Recommended Time Frames,* Apr. 2009. http://www.gao.gov/new.items/d09347.pdf (accessed Jul. 15, 2009).

2. Institute for Healthcare Improvement: *Improving Flow Through Acute Care Settings.* http://www.ihi.org/IHI/Programs/Collaboratives/ImprovingFlow ThroughAcuteCareSettings.htm (accessed Jul. 15, 2009).

3. The Joint Commission: *2009 Comprehensive Accreditation Manual for Hospitals: The Official Handbook.* Oakbrook Terrace, IL: Joint Commission Resources, 2008.

4. Litvak E.: Optimizing patient flow by managing its variability. In *Front Office to Front Line: Essential Issues for Health Care Leaders.* Oakbrook Terrace, IL: Joint Commission Resources, 2005, pp. 91–111.

5. Healthcare Financial Management Association: *How Hospitals Are Combating the Financial Downturn. Healthcare Financial Pulse,* Apr. 2009. http://www.hfma.org/NR/rdonlyres/B5FE7CAD-6BC4-449C-BA21-08D170F5B28C/0/Pulse.pdf (accessed Jul. 15, 2009).

6. Litvak E., et al.: Managing unnecessary variability in patient demand to reduce nursing stress and improve patient safety. *Jt Comm J Qual Patient Saf* 31:330–338, Jun. 2005.

7. Personal communication between author and Joan Massella, R.N., M.Ed., M.B.A., administrative vice president and chief nursing officer, St. Clair Hospital, Mt. Lebanon, Pennsylvania, Jun. 26, 2009.

8. The Joint Commission: *Facts About the Tracer Methodology.* http://www. jointcommission.org/AboutUs/Fact_Sheets/Tracer_Methodology.htm (accessed Jun. 24, 2009).

9. McManus M.L., et al.: Variability in surgical caseload and access to intensive care services. *Anesthesiology* 98:1491–1496, Jun. 2003.

10. Institute of Medicine: *To Err Is Human: Building a Safer Health System.* Washington, DC: National Academy Press, 2000.

11. Rogers A.E., et al.: The working hours of hospital staff nurses and patient safety. *Health Aff (Millwood)* 23:202–212, Jul./Aug. 2004.

12. Personal communication between author and Deborah J. Kaczynski, M.S., administrative director, Ancillary Services & Capacity Management, University of Pittsburgh Medical Center (Mercy), Feb. 2009.

13. Personal communication between author and David Kish, B.A., R.N., C.C.R.N., executive director, Emergency Services and Patient Logistics, St. Clair Hospital, Mt. Lebanon, PA, Jun. 25, 2009.

14. The Joint Commission: Case Study: Reducing overcrowding in the ED with the full capacity protocol. *Joint Commission Benchmark* 11:3–4, Jul./Aug. 2009.

15. Litvak E., McManus M.L., Cooper A.: A Root Cause Analysis of Emergency Department Crowding and Ambulance Diversion in Massachusetts. *Boston University Program for the Management of Variability in Health Care Delivery, Report to the Massachusetts Department of Public Health,* Oct. 2002. http://www.mass.gov/Eeohhs2/docs/dph/quality/healthcare/ad_emergency_dept_analysis.doc (accessed Jul. 1, 2009).

16. Glowers M.M.: *Left Without Being Seen.* http://www.hgexperts.com/article. asp?id=6067 (accessed Jul. 15, 2009).

17. Nawar E.W., Niska R.W., Xu J.: *National Hospital Ambulatory Medical Care Survey: 2005 Emergency Department Summary,* Jun. 07. http://cdc.gov/nchs/data/ad/ad386.pdf (accessed Jul. 1, 2009).

18. U.S. General Accountability Office (GAO): *Emergency Departments: Crowded Conditions Vary Among Hospitals and Communities,* Mar. 2003 (accessed Jul. 15, 2009).

19. Falvo T., et al.: The financial impact of ambulance diversions and patient elopements. *Acad Emerg Med* 14:58–62, Jan. 2007.

20. McConnell K.J., Richards C.F., Daya M.: Ambulance diversion and lost hospital revenues. *Ann Emerg Med* 48:702–710, Dec. 2006. Epub Jul. 11, 2006.

21. Blewett D.: LGH surgery patients waiting for ICU beds. *The Examiner,* Jun. 26, 2009. http://www.examiner.com.au/news/local/news/health/surgery-patients-wait-for-icu-beds-19-elective-cases-cancelled-in-mayjune/1551292.aspx (accessed Jul. 2, 2009).

22. Dexter F., et al.: Validation of statistical methods to compare cancellation rates on the day of surgery. *Anesth Analg* 101:465–473, Aug. 2005.

23. Park K.W.: *Scope of Operating Room Cancellations for a Busy University Hospital Vascular Surgical Service* [abstract]. American Society of Anesthesiologists Annual Meeting, Orlando, FL, Oct. 18–22, 2008. http://www.asaabstracts.com/strands/asaabstracts/abstract.htm;jsessionid=716C1002FCBC0C61B16D8B96 07B4B5D3?year=2002&index=13&absnum=380 (accessed Jul. 2, 2009).

24. Kobis D.A., Kennedy K.M.: Capacity management and patient throughput: Putting this problem to bed. *Healthc Financ Manage* 60:88–92, 94, Oct. 2006.

25. Personal communication between author and Lucy Shoupp, R.N., M.S.H.A., administrative vice president, chief quality officer, St. Clair Hospital, Mt. Lebanon, PA, Jul. 9, 2009.

Chapter 2

Impact of Patient Flow Issues on Nursing Staff and Patients

Peter I. Buerhaus, Ph.D., R.N., F.A.A.N.; Anne Miller, Ph.D., R.N.

"When a CEO says to me, 'What's the business case for safety?, I do not say to them what I am thinking, which is, 'You clearly do not get it, because obviously safety *is* our business'[1(p. 370)]

Hospital managers, physicians, nurses, and many others work together to provide high-quality and safe patient care. Each performs different work, is guided by a unique disciplinary perspective, and carries out his or her responsibilities within a complex and rapidly changing environment. Clinicians focus on providing individualized patient care, while managers seek to improve facilities and systems of care, provide resources, and ensure an overall environment that supports the patient-centered activities of clinicians. The quality and safety of patient care and hospitals' ability to operate efficiently and manage stressors depend on effective coordination, communication, and problem solving among and between these groups.

As Chapter 1 makes clear, poorly controlled patient flow is an important stressor. The teamwork, communication, and problem solving needed to manage surges in patient census and minimize their impact require that hospital decision makers first recognize that poorly controlled patient flow is a problem that profoundly affects hospital managers, nurses, and patients. Increases in patient admissions can overwhelm managers and nursing staff and create temporary shortages of nurses, potentially jeopardizing care quality and safety. Although there is evidence that hospitals have responded to the current nursing shortage by improving characteristics of their clinical environment,[2] a recent study showed wide variation in hospital executives', physicians', and nurses' perceptions of the effects of the nursing shortage* on patient care quality, safety, and professional relationships.[3]

The purpose of this chapter is to increase hospital decision makers' recognition of the effects of poorly controlled patient flow. It focuses on understanding how patient flow affects the three levels of the organization most directly involved in ensuring that surges in patient demand do not compromise care delivery and patient outcomes: unit area supervision, unit management, and nursing staff. We illustrate these impacts by providing a vignette that depicts how a "typical" nursing supervisor, unit manager, and nurse respond to both planned and unplanned changes in patient flow. The decisions, problem solving, and challenges that each

---

* However, the effect of the current economy on the nursing shortage is discussed later (see page 23).

level experiences when implementing adaptive response strategies are critical to the effectiveness, quality, and safety of a hospital's care delivery systems. We then review the published research literature on the relationship between hospital nurse staffing and patient outcomes, including variability in patient census and its impact on nurses' workload, and the potential that patients might not be receiving needed nursing care. We then examine changes in the nursing workforce that are expected to negatively affect the physical capacity of many nurses and restrict the future size of the workforce. We conclude the chapter by describing the benefits that can be expected when hospital management acts to control peaks in patient flow.

Vignette Depicting Impact of Patient Flow

To understand the effects of patient flow, it is important to consider the physical and cognitive work that nurses undertake to manage fluctuations in patient census arising from natural (uncontrollable) variability contributed by the emergency department (ED) and the artificial (potentially controllable and thus unnecessary) peaks of patient flow into the hospital arising principally from elective operations. As Miller and Xiao[4] observed, decisions about patient admissions are made at multiple, interconnected levels of management. Thus, in the following vignette we describe the effects of variability in patient flow from the perspective of a hypothetical nursing supervisor, charge nurse, and nurse in an acute care hospital. The vignette illustrates the information gathering and deciphering, decision making, reprioritizing, and unexpected challenges that each level confronts and how decisions at one level affect the decisions and actions made by management and clinicians at other levels. Although the individuals represented in our vignettes are fictitious, their experiences are based in part on observations gleaned from ethnographic studies of care coordination.[5,6]

Nursing Supervisor's Perspective

Helen arrives at the hospital early to prepare for the morning handoff (handover) report. She works at a medium-sized community hospital that operates several residency programs in conjunction with a major medical center 35 miles away, in the center of a large city. Helen manages nursing resources and bed allocation for 4 medical and 4 surgical units. She is one of four supervisors who manage 24 units, the ED, operating room (OR), and 2 ICUs. Helen logs into the hospital bed-management computer system and proceeds to the ED, where she learns that there are no emergency patients, but six nonurgent patients are waiting to be seen. While typical for a Thursday morning, if this were Sunday morning, there would likely be several emergency patients

and double the number of patients in the waiting room. Helen notes that the same two patients (both with pneumonia) who were waiting for a bed when she left the hospital yesterday are still waiting to be transferred to a nursing unit. Although they do their best to turn these patients frequently to prevent skin breakdown and promote pulmonary ventilation (to prevent atelectasis), it is difficult for ED nurses to provide high-quality care to sick patients lying on gurneys.

Helen checks the status of her medical and surgical units and observes that little has changed since yesterday—even 92-year-old Mrs. Jones, who was not expected to survive the night, is still alive. Helen writes a note to remind herself to find out if any progress has been made to arrange beds in local long-term facilities needed by the four medical patients whom she expects will be discharged today. She also realizes that five surgical unit patients are expected to be discharged today. The surgical discharges will not help the ED patients but will free beds for the weekend influx of patients arriving through the ED. Helen knows that case managers, social workers, unit charge nurses, and unit nurses will need to coordinate their efforts to organize all the patient transfers during the day, particularly with the weekend drawing near.

Helen also checks the surgical schedule. On Thursdays, the surgeons usually try to perform as many outpatient operations as possible before the weekend. Four of the eight ORs are allocated for orthopedic and plastic surgery elective in- and outpatient procedures, three rooms are open for short cases and emergencies, and one OR is closed because of a shortage of nursing staff. Helen notes that each OR schedule includes patients who are on "standby" in case scheduled procedures are cancelled or there is time for additional procedures before 5:00 P.M. (17:00). The list for one of the surgeons, who has a reputation for trying to conduct as many surgeries as she can, is very long. Although this benefits patients by reducing their wait time, and the "extra volume" increases hospital revenues, complications sometimes develop during surgery, or patients do not recover as quickly or safely as expected and cannot be discharged. When this occurs, additional work is created for hospital staff, who must find beds for these unplanned admissions.

Next, Helen reviews nurse staffing for the day shift. Although it is only 6:15 A.M. (06:15), five nurses have already called in sick, and Helen knows from experience that it will be another hour before she has a complete absentee count. She also knows that there were eight nurses available in the hospital's temporary staffing pool and another five from temporary staffing agencies. Five of the pool nurses have already been called in to cover the absentees, leaving eight nurses in reserve. However, Helen realizes that this is not a true indicator of availability because one pool nurse is a midwife, two are ICU nurses, and one nurse refuses to work on a surgical unit, thereby limiting Helen's ability to match nurses with the appropriate experience and skills to the units that can best use them. Beyond the day shift, there are nine vacancies to fill for the Thursday night shift, so even if additional surgical cases can be admitted during the day, there may not be enough staff to care for these patients overnight. There are also gaps in Friday's schedule. Looking ahead to the weekend, Helen expects that it is going to be difficult to balance patient demand with available beds and the number and type of nurses required.

Having gained this broad overview, Helen joins the three other supervisors for the night supervisors' report. The night supervisors confirm Helen's assessment that the two ED patients need to be transferred to a nursing unit, but this cannot happen until patients are discharged. With respect to the units under Helen's supervision, the night supervisor notes that Mrs. Jones's condition has deteriorated substantially during the past hour and that her family has been summoned to the hospital. Furthermore, a patient suffered a probable stroke and might die within the day. After much discussion with family members, another patient has agreed to accept a bed in a nursing home, which may mean that the patient will be discharged sometime today. Each of these situations could result in an available bed, but each requires great sensitivity to the needs of patients and their loved ones. It seems likely, however, that the two ED patients will be able to occupy a hospital bed later in the day. The unit charge nurses will need to be informed about the transferring ED patients. Shaking her head, the night supervisor also makes sure that everyone is aware of the all-too-familiar bloated size of the OR waiting list. Before the report is completed, another three nurses have called in sick, and Helen hopes that their respective charge nurses are checking with their staff to find someone willing to work an extra shift. Helen telephones the hospital staffing pool coordinator and two temporary staffing agencies and requests three nurses to staff her units.

At the night supervisors' departure at 7:30 A.M. (07:30), Helen learns that Mrs. Jones has just died. The charge nurse wants to know whether there are any nurses who could be spared for 30 to 45 minutes to care for the other patients to whom Mrs. Jones's nurse is assigned; the charge nurse wants Mrs. Jones's nurse to focus on attending to the family's needs. Helen calls the charge nurse to ascertain the needs of the other patients assigned to Mrs. Jones's nurse and is told that both patients require help with their breakfast. Helen scans her staff list and notes that one of her units has two licensed practical nurses (L.P.N.s). She calls the charge nurse and explains the situation, and one of the L.P.N.s is sent to temporarily relieve Mrs. Jones's nurse.

It was raining when she drove to work, and so Helen is not surprised when at 8:45 A.M. (08:45) her pager notifies her that two automobile accident patients are being airlifted to the ED in critical condition and four more are arriving by ambulance. Helen knows that the ED and ORs have been paged and that their respective on-call staff members have been summoned. Transferring the two ED medical patients with pneumonia is now a priority because the ED nurses will be needed to receive the emergency patients. She wishes that the elective surgery list were shorter and hopes that nothing goes wrong that would result in additional admissions.

Helen calls the medical unit case manager to find out when the nursing home patient can be transferred. She then walks to the medical unit to see the patient herself and to talk with the charge nurse about the unit's staffing. Next, she assesses the situation involving Mrs. Jones and learns that to the relief of family, Mrs. Jones died peacefully. Because the nurse taking care of Mrs. Jones was able to help the family, they have left the hospital and are on their way to make funeral arrangements. The charge nurse is currently waiting for housekeeping staff to clean Mrs. Jones's hospital room and informs Helen that the surgical fellow just called from the OR, requesting a bed for a postsurgical outpatient who appears to have suffered a cardiac event in the recovery room. The patient is currently in the cardiac catheterization laboratory but will need to be monitored for 24 hours. Mrs. Jones was in a monitored bed, and her former nurse is competent in reading and interpreting cardiac telemetry. Helen must now balance the ED patient's need for a bed against the recovery room patient's needs. She pages her colleague to determine whether the ED patient might be accommodated in one of the other units but learns that another night-shift nurse has just called in sick and that the charge nurse is reluctant to receive any more patients, given her unit's current staffing level and skill mix. For Helen, this means that three additional pool or agency nurses will be needed for the night shift. Helen also realizes that, excluding the charge nurse, only one of the nurses working on the night shift is familiar with the unit's operations and nursing staff and with the nursing needs of patients. Helen is beginning to worry about the safety of the patients on this unit during the upcoming night shift.

Helen proceeds to check on the two other surgical units that she is assigned to supervise. She is not concerned about the patients who have been airlifted to the ED because, if they survive, they will be admitted directly to currently vacant beds in the ICUs. However, Helen is concerned about the four patients arriving by ambulance. Five surgical patients were identified as possible discharges pending approval from the surgical fellow. Three of the patients are in one unit and two in a second. Two nurses who work on the first unit called in sick, and that unit also has two nurses missing from the night shift. The second unit also had two nurses go home sick, and Helen doubts that they will return to work tonight. Helen sighs as she accepts that gaps in the schedule, particularly the night shift, result from the hospital's ongoing inability to recruit nurses to fill open positions.

A Charge Nurse's Perspective

Mark is the day-shift charge nurse managing one of Helen's 20-bed surgical units. Mark is concerned with finding staff willing to fill gaps in the night shift and tomorrow's day shift. Currently, he needs three nurses to cover the night shift and two for the day shift. Mark cannot remember the last time the night shift was fully staffed by nurses who worked permanently on the unit. One staff member, Leroy, is on call, and Mark telephones him early so that Leroy can plan his day, knowing that he will be working tonight. There is no point in calling the night-shift nurses to ask if they might work an extra shift because they are now home and sleeping. Mark could leave phone messages but knows that personal requests are more successful. (He sometimes uses his wife's cell phone to call staff because they know his telephone number, and some nurses will not talk with him if they recognize Mark's number.)

Two of the surgical teams have already conducted patient rounds on Mark's unit, and the night-shift charge nurse reported that up to four patients might be going home today. Discharging a patient is as time-consuming as admitting a patient. Patients and their families need education about how they are going to manage at home, questions about their medications need to be answered, transportation needs to be arranged, and a number of other needs may arise. After the patient has left the unit, housekeeping needs to clean the room and bed as soon as possible. Of the five possible discharges, only three were approved for discharge during the surgical rounds. Because one patient spiked a temperature and a second complained of pain, the surgical team decided to postpone discharges for an additional day. While rounding, the surgical fellow received a message that two patients were arriving in the ED by helicopter and will need to be assessed for possible surgery. Moreover, the fellow learned that four additional patients were on their way to the ED by ambulance. As he was leaving for the ED, the fellow asked Mark for the unit's bed status and was told that the unit could admit three patients after the discharged patients' rooms had been cleaned.

Mark decides that he needs to personally assess the three patients awaiting discharge. The first patient is a young man who had been involved in a motorbike accident and suffered serious leg fractures and soft-tissue trauma. His fractures have been set, but he has a wound that requires frequent dressing changes. During the past few days the patient has dressed his wounds under

nursing supervision and has walked safely using crutches. His sister will arrive at the hospital within the hour to transport him home. The second patient presents a similarly uncomplicated scenario. Anticipating that some of the patients arriving to the ED are likely to be admitted, Mark instructs the patients' nurses to call housekeeping as soon as each patient has left his or her room. The nurses of both discharged patients take this as an indicator that they are likely to be assigned a new patient later in the shift, although this has not been confirmed. The third patient to be discharged is an older man with a new colostomy. He is physically able to go home, but his nurse and the stomatherapy team are concerned that the patient and his wife have not demonstrated that they are ready to properly manage the colostomy, despite several days of instruction and practice. The patient's wife is coming in to take her husband home, but Mark does not know whether this will be in the morning or afternoon. Mark, the patient's nurse, and the stomatherapy nurse decide to involve the patient and his wife in an intensive training session. Mark makes a mental note to check whether the case manager has arranged for a home health nurse to work with the family at home.

Helen arrives to discuss bed availability and staffing levels. Mark informs her that two patients are about to go home and a third will probably be discharged later but, unexpectedly, two patients will not be going home today. Mark explains that the day-shift nurse discovered that one patient had spiked a temperature. Despite the patient reporting that he told the temporary agency nurse that he did not feel well, his temperature was not taken during the night. Although the agency nurse had done his best, this was his first time on this unit, and he had focused his attention on two patients who were more acutely ill. Helen and Mark bemoan the difficulties associated with having fewer permanently employed night nurses; they have had this discussion many times.

Mark also informs Helen that the surgical fellow mentioned that accident victims are arriving in the ED. Mark and Helen review the unit's staffing needs for the next two shifts. Fortunately, Leroy confirmed that he will work tonight. Mark lists the other staff members he has telephoned and says that he does not expect to hear from them until after 5:00 P.M. (17:00), if at all. Mark also notes that two recently hired new graduates have the day off. Although both are enthusiastic and willing to help the unit, Mark and Helen want to guard against the long-term risks of burnout and agree that they will not call them unless all other options to secure staff fail. Until the surgical team decides whether to admit any of the ED arrivals, Mark will make sure that rooms are cleaned, restocked, and ready for patients. Helen will request staff from the hospital pool coordinator and temporary staffing agencies. Helen hopes for the best but knows that it is not always possible to get pool nurses to agree to work the needed shift.

Two hours later, the surgical fellow notifies Mark that one of the accident victims, a 52-year-old man, is being taken to the OR for treatment of abdominal injuries. The procedure should take about two hours but might take longer. Mark calls Helen to confirm the new patient's admission and to inquire about additional staff for the night shift and tomorrow's day shift. He then checks his list of patients and nursing staff to determine the most appropriate bed for this patient, given other patients on the unit and the nurses' workload. On his unit, most nurses care for between four and six patients, but this can vary, depending on patient needs and availability of nursing staff. Mark tries to balance the workload for his staff so that each nurse has no more than one relatively sick patient at any time, along with several less acutely ill patients. Mark also considers the potential for cross-infection between patients, a patient's age and gender, and the needs and disposition of families. Mark decides that the new patient is best located in the bed occupied by the colostomy patient and places a telephone call to ascertain the outcome of the colostomy instruction session.

A Nurse's Perspective

Sue has been working on the surgical unit for nearly three years. Today she is caring for five patients, including Mr. Taylor, who has Parkinson's disease and is having difficulty managing his new colostomy. During the past three days Sue and the stomatherapist have been working with Mr. Taylor and his wife to increase their confidence and ability to take care of his colostomy. Sue and the Taylors are aiming for discharge today. Sue's other patients include Ms. Jackson, who was admitted yesterday with newly diagnosed Type 2 diabetes; Mr. Williams, a young man recovering from removal of a ruptured appendix; and two patients recovering from abdominal surgery, one of whom requires considerable wound care.

As Sue and the stomatherapy nurse are finishing the session with Mr. and Mrs. Taylor, Mark enters the room to assess Mr. Taylor's readiness for discharge. Mrs. Taylor says with great delight that this is the first time they have changed the bag and dressed the stoma without spilling anything. The stomatherapist relates that the stoma and surrounding skin is clean and pink and that she believes that Mr. Taylor is ready for discharge. Sue has already packed stoma supplies for the weekend and reassures the Taylors that the home health nurse will visit on Monday. She also reviews Mr. Taylor's medications to be sure that he and his wife understand what they are for and when to take them; she then completes the hospital's discharge checklist. After Sue says goodbye to the Taylors, Mark tells Sue that she will receive a new patient from the OR in two hours or maybe less.

Sue scans her medication and tasks list. Now her most immediate priorities are to change Mrs. Ramirez's dressing, test Ms. Jackson's blood glucose, and administer intravenous (IV) antibiotics scheduled at 12:00 noon (12:00) for James with the ruptured appendix. Mrs. Ramirez's dressing is time-consuming because she is disoriented, does not speak English, and becomes quite anxious. Sue knows that Mrs. Ramirez's daughter is expected at around 12:30 P.M. (12:30) for lunch and that Mrs. Ramirez is much calmer when her daughter is present for the dressing. Sue decides to give Mr. Williams's antibiotic before taking Ms. Jackson's blood glucose. This will allow her to spend time talking with Ms. Jackson about her diabetes, particularly to assess her knowledge about the disease and how she is coping emotionally. After administering the IV antibiotic to Mr. Williams, Sue checks her notes and is reminded that the dietitian has already spoken to Ms. Jackson this morning. Rather than overwhelm her with more information, Sue asks Ms. Jackson whether she has any questions about her diabetes. Ms. Jackson bursts into tears and says that her grandmother had diabetes and sobs, "Her leg went black, and she had to have it amputated." As Sue draws a curtain to provide privacy, Mark enters the room and tells Sue that her emergency patient's procedure has finished earlier than expected and that the patient is now in the recovery room and will be coming to the unit in about 30 minutes. Mark also says that the patient's wife and son are in the visitors' room and that he has oriented them to the unit, explained visiting hour policies, and told them to expect to meet with Sue in the next few minutes.

Sue realizes she must reorganize her plans to accommodate the new-patient admission. She briefly tells Mark about Ms. Jackson's concern and asks him to check the room for the new patient to ensure that needed equipment is present and operational. She also mentions that Mrs. Ramirez's wound needs to be dressed but that her daughter has not yet arrived and that she is concerned that Mrs. Ramirez's dressing may be delayed. Mark suggests that Sue prepare the dressing materials and that if Sue is unable to complete the dressing before the new patient arrives, then if possible he will arrange for someone else to help. Sue returns to Ms. Jackson's and reiterates some of the dietitian's key messages: "Yes, diabetes has complications, but with a weight control plan, proper diet, and exercise, complications can be minimized." Sue explains that one of the reasons Ms. Jackson is in the hospital is so that they can develop a plan for her to manage her diabetes successfully. Thankfully, Ms. Jackson seems consoled. Sue pages the dietitian, recounts her conversation with Ms. Jackson, and suggests that a visit from one of the diabetes support group members might be a good idea.

As Sue finishes collecting Mrs. Ramirez's dressing materials, recovery room staff suddenly appear, wheeling her new patient onto the unit. The recovery room nurse gives her report, and Sue completes a full assessment and physical examination of Mr. Angelo, the 52-year-old man involved in the automobile accident earlier today. Sue checks his abdominal dressings and drain tubes, as well as the surgeon's orders and Mr. Angelo's medication and IV fluid orders. Mr. Angelo is still sleepy and says he feels nauseated; something about his demeanor makes Sue feel uneasy. Sue discovers that the room has not been stocked with an emesis basin and, while walking to the supply room, she stops in Ms. Jackson's room and finds that her IV fluid bag is empty. If Sue does not act fast, a clot will form in the vein, and a new IV will have to be inserted. Sue looks for someone to cross-check Ms. Jackson's IV solution to verify that it is the right medication for the right patient, but the nurses looking after the patient next to Ms. Jackson are too busy to stop and help her. Wanting to check on Mr. Angelo, Sue leaves Ms. Jackson's room, deciding that her IV will have to wait. As she returns to Mr. Angelo's bed she passes the visitor's room, introduces herself to Mr. Angelo's wife and son, and gives them a summary of his condition.

On entering Mr. Angelo's room, Sue is startled to find him vomiting a large volume of bright red blood. Sue pulls the curtains and asks a nearby nurse to page the surgical fellow. Mark observes the sudden bustle and investigates, saying that the fellow has gone to the OR to assess the second of the accident victims who will also be admitted to the unit. Staying with Mr. Angelo, Sue asks again whether anyone can change Mrs. Ramirez's dressing, and Mark relates that the other nurses are too busy at the moment. Sue stays with Mr. Angelo to help him stay as calm as possible, assesses his skin color and respirations, takes his blood pressure, and checks his pulse for any signs of hypovolemic shock. Mark has taken Mr. Angelo's wife and son back to the waiting room and tells them that a physician has been called to check on him.

Sue's shift has nearly passed, and the night-shift staff will be arriving in one hour. Mr. Angelo is still vomiting blood and will probably return to the OR. Ms. Jackson's IV was finally restarted. However, Mrs. Ramirez's dressing has not been changed, and her daughter is agitated and unhappy with Sue. Sue has not started to update her charting. She knows that she will not be leaving work on time and will miss her son's first soccer practice and that her daughter needs to be picked up from day care. She calls her husband, who, although annoyed, agrees to pick up the children and bring home dinner from a fast-food restaurant. Sue calculates how much her paycheck will increase because of the overtime she is about to work but sighs because she would rather spend that time with her family.

Comments

Regardless of their position, each of the nurses portrayed in this vignette, which describes the experiences of individuals representing the three levels of the hospital who are directly involved in responding to changes in patient census, began his or her shift by assessing the overall state of the unit(s) or patients for whom he or she is responsible. This assessment included estimating the expected demand for hospital beds, determining the current and future availability of nursing staff, and becoming aware of the specific demands of patients and their families. Each of the nurses—Helen, Mark, and Sue—then prioritized his or her workload, anticipated future needs, and planned for contingencies that might be put into place to accommodate the unexpected. The quality and safety of patient care and the hospital's ability to operate efficiently while managing the stress created by surges in patient demand depends on effective coordination, communication, and problem solving among and between the nursing supervisor, unit manager, and nurse providing direct patient care.

This vignette provides a glimpse of some of the activities, people, and decisions that might take place when there is an unanticipated increase in patient census. We ignored other discussion among other supervisors, charge nurses, and numerous nursing staff who were affected by and responded to the influx of patients. In addition, we left untold the effect of decisions that may or may not have resulted in new problems for both nurses and patients. For example, what happened to the two ED medical patients? Were they transferred to a unit, or did their delay result in a worsening of their condition and admission to the ICU with respiratory failure? How many of the surgeon's elective OR patients were unexpectedly admitted to units, and what were the consequences? Were enough nurses found to staff the upcoming night shift? Did the 52-year-old accident victim go into shock, did he require surgery, or was he transferred to an ICU? Were all medications given on time and to the right patients? Given all the events of this day, it is not unreasonable to suspect that some patients were at increased risk for adverse outcomes during their hospitalization.

Each of the nurses in the vignette was operating in a boundary between safe and unsafe and between high and low quality of care. Working on the boundary of safe and unsafe practice is inherently risky as it involves making choices between truly good practice and compromised practice, even if the compromise is only marginal.[7] As Amalberti and colleagues[8] observe, the more frequently compromised practice occurs, the more likely it is to be accepted as the norm.

Nurse Staffing, Variability in Patient Admissions, and Patient Outcomes

Whether planned or unscheduled, the arrival of new patients on a nursing unit changes the workload of nurses. The change in workload depends on the number of new patients the nurse is assigned and the clinical needs of the patient (as well as the needs of family). In addition, as illustrated in the vignette, changes in patient flow increase the cognitive work of supervisors, unit managers, and nurses. But how is the quality of patient care affected when workload changes? More precisely, are patients at increased risk for lower quality and unsafe care when nursing staff contend with surges in patient demand? This section addresses these questions by reviewing the published literature on the relationship between hospital nurse staffing and patient outcomes, examining short-term variability of patient admissions on patient outcomes, and summarizing recent results on missed patient care by nurses.

Until the latter part of the 1990s, credible evidence of the relationship of hospital nurse staffing and patient outcomes was sorely lacking. As managed care spread during the early 1990s, nurses complained that the number of patients assigned per nurse was increasing at the same time that hospitalized patients were more acutely ill and length of stay was decreasing. As hospitals attempted to lower their costs to survive in an increasingly competitive environment, many reduced the support staff that assisted nurses with indirect patient care activities. Nurses believed that these responses resulted in a deterioration of the quality and safety of patient care and voiced their concerns loudly and often. The U.S. Congress and the Secretary of Health and Human Services responded by requesting that the Institute of Medicine (IOM) undertake a study to investigate nurse staffing in hospitals and other organizations. The IOM report *Nurse Staffing in Hospitals and Nursing Homes: Is It Adequate?*[9] examined a wide range of issues involving hospital staffing levels but reported a paucity of evidence on the relationship between nurse staffing and adverse patient outcomes. The IOM committee recommended that research be conducted to address this issue. This recommendation, spurred by the growth of the quality improvement movement and the publication of the IOM's report *To Err Is Human*,[10] resulted in a rapid increase in the number of studies investigating this relationship.

The studies we summarize reflect a variety of data sources and different measures of patient outcomes and nurse staffing and are based on the hospital, nursing unit, and patient levels of analysis. Patient outcomes have been constructed from relatively inexpensive and publicly available administrative data (typically hospital discharge abstracts), which yield large samples of cases for analysis; and from medical charts, which, through a more expensive

process, have to be collected and abstracted and which usually result in smaller samples for analysis. In general, studies tend to focus on either medical or surgical patients (but rarely both) and often exclude pediatric, obstetric, emergency, and inpatient psychiatric patients. Data to measure nurse staffing typically come from special state surveys; investigator-initiated surveys; national data such as the American Hospital Association or the Agency for Healthcare Quality and Research Health Care Utilization National Inpatient Sample; or individual nursing units and hospitals. Published studies have attempted to account for hospital differences by controlling for hospital characteristics such as teaching or community status, technology, location, and ownership. In addition, researchers have attempted to control for differences in the patient severity of illness and have used a variety of analytic methods to test for relationships.

Inpatient Nurse Staffing and Patient Complications

Studies report an inverse relationship between nurse staffing (usually unspecified as either number of nurses or patient-to-nurse ratio [PNR]) and patient complications. For example, nurse staffing has been found to be associated with hospital-acquired nosocomial infections,[11–13] sepsis and bloodstream infections,[14–17] pneumonia,[15,18–21] falls,[22–24] urinary tract infections,[18,19,25,26] upper gastrointestinal bleeding,[18] medication errors,[22,26] shock and cardiac arrest,[18] pressure ulcers,[21,25,26] and longer-than-expected length of stay.[11,14,18, 20,24,25]

Studies have also examined the association between higher nurse staffing levels and decreased mortality but have reached mixed conclusions. A study by Needleman and colleagues[18] that was based on more than 6 million discharges from 799 hospitals in 11 U.S. states, showed an inverse relationship between nurse staffing levels and "failure to rescue," defined in that study as death among patients who had one of five complications (pneumonia, sepsis, shock or cardiac arrest, upper gastrointestinal bleeding, or deep vein thrombosis) in surgical patients and to a lesser extent in medical patients. A study of 168 Pennsylvania hospitals conducted by Aiken and colleagues[27] reported that after adjusting for patient and hospital characteristics, each additional patient per nurse added above the specified optimal staffing ratio of one nurse per four patients calculated in this study was associated with a 7% increase in the likelihood of dying within 30 days of admission and a 7% increase in the odds of failure to rescue. Other studies have found an association between nurse staffing and hospital mortality.[28–31] In addition, in a study of neonatal patient outcomes, Hamilton et al.[32] reported that risk-adjusted mortality was reduced by 48% in two-thirds of understaffed neonatal ICUs as the ratio of registered nurses (R.N.s) with neonatal qualifications for high-risk infants to patients reached one to one. However, other studies have not found an association between nurse staffing and mortality in adult patients.[33–35]

Although these studies provide evidence that hospital nurse staffing levels matter to the quality of patient care, they do not examine how staffing levels change over time, the reasons they change, and potential effect on patients. As the vignette suggests, nurses' workload changes as patients flow into and out of the hospital, the severity of patients' illnesses changes, or staffing increases of decreases (adding to or subtracting from the number of patients assigned to each nurse). The studies now examined focus on determining the extent of short-term variability in hospital admissions, the sources of this variability, how frequently and how much nurse workloads change, and impact on patient outcomes.

Short-Term Variability in Patient Admissions

Researchers have examined the extent of short-term variability in the volume of hospital admissions, the sources of such variability, and the potential link to instability in hospital census. For example, Litvak and colleagues[36,37] describe the sources of variable patient admissions and emphasize the importance of day-to-day fluctuations in the volumes of scheduled admissions. Other studies report a connection between the number of scheduled (elective) admissions and ED overcrowding, ambulance diversions, efficiency of the surgical department, quality of patient care, stress on hospital staff, and diversions from a pediatric ICU (PICU).[38–42] Although a limited body of research has been conducted, evidence suggests that short-term variability in patient admissions affects nurses' workload. For example, Budreau and colleagues[43] reported hourly variability in the number of nursing hours per patient day (HPPD) and in the PNR in several units in one hospital. The variability in the PNR measured on an hourly basis was found to be substantially greater than when the PNR was measured on a daily basis. Another study documented how PNR in an ED varied over one half-hour periods, from 0.5 to 9.0 patients per nurse, with a mean of 3.5.[44] Others have documented variability in the PNR (or similar staffing measures) during longer units of time, including shift to shift,[45–47] day to day,[17,46,48–53] week to week,[54] and monthly.[13,16]

Studies reported in the critical care medicine, hospital epidemiology, and nursing literatures suggest that short-term variability in staffing levels is associated with the variety and number of adverse patient outcomes. Studies of intensive care and burn units report that temporary decreases in nurse staffing were linked to increases in nosocomial infections,[13,51,55] mortality rates,[56,57] bloodstream infections,[16,17] infections with methicillin-resistant *Staphylococcus aureus* (MRSA),[48,49,54,58–61] infections from other organisms,[13,50,62–64] and ventilator-associated pneumonia.[52] Ream

and colleagues[45] reported that the likelihood of an unplanned extubation in a PICU was 3.8 times higher in shifts where nurse workloads, adjusted for census and patient severity measured by patient acuity level (PAL), exceeded 6.3 PALs, compared with shifts with PALs lower than 5. Similarly, Haley and Bregman[48] reported that the odds ratio for clusters of staphylococcal infections in a neonatal special care unit was 16 times higher after patient exposures to PNR that exceeded 7, which was viewed as a critical threshold level, compared with lower PNRs. In contrast, in a more recent study, Evans and Kim[65] found no association in peaks of admissions with patient mortality; however, because they did not directly measure either patient census or staffing levels, the ability to determine an association of PNR with patient outcomes was limited.

Missed-Nursing-Care and Systemic Impacts

We conclude this section of the review of the literature by summarizing a recent study that sought to identify the nursing care that is actually being delivered to patients. Kalisch and colleagues,[66] who surveyed 459 R.N.s in 28 inpatient units across three hospitals, found that patient assessments were reported missed (by 44% of the R.N. respondents), nursing interventions and basic care were missed (73%), and planning nursing care was missed (71%). The six most frequently missed nursing activities were ambulating patients (reported by 84% of the R.N.s), assessing effectiveness of medications (83%), turning patients (82%), providing oral care (82%), teaching (80%), and administering PRN ("as needed") medications (80%). As noted by the colleagues, the omission of several of these nursing activities has been associated with adverse patient outcomes. For example, failure to ambulate and turn patients is linked to delirium,[67] pneumonia,[68] increased length of stay and delayed discharge,[69–71] increased pain and discomfort,[72] and physical disability.[73] The authors reported that the most cited reason for missed care pertained to the lack of labor:

> The critical element in this category was not levels of staffing per se (although it was also reported to be problematic) but the unplanned increases in demand for patient care in both volume and acuity.[66(p. 7)]

In addition, inadequate supplies, including medications, were reported to be a major issue, and communication breakdowns were reported by 25% to 51% of respondents.[66]

Finally, Pedroja[74] conducted a study that used different measures of patient volume and examined incident reports filed by hospital staff in two hospitals in a 515-day period. The exploratory study demonstrated that increased volume was related to increased medical errors with serious harm to patients, including death.

Moreover, the study documented that beyond nursing units, other hospital departments (for example, laboratory, pharmacy, radiology, housekeeping, and engineering) are overwhelmed, pulled in multiple directions, and unable to keep up with requests from those providing direct patient care.

Taken as a whole, an increasing body of evidence indicates that inadequate hospital nurse staffing is associated with an increased risk of adverse patient outcomes. Although the underlying processes behind this linkage are not well understood, variations in patient census and surges in patient demand can affect nurse workload and in turn are likely to increase the risk of adverse outcomes and complications. Failing to provide needed nursing care to patients may be a consequence of surges in demand.

Emerging Problems in the Nursing Workforce

In the previous section, we addressed why we should be concerned about the impact of poorly controlled patient flow on nurses by examining research on the relationship between hospital nurse staffing and patient complications, including mortality, missed nursing care, and impact of short-term variability in hospital admissions on nursing workload. Clearly, there is reason to be concerned that continuing with existing processes for handling patient flow, particularly surges in patient demand, is likely to overwhelm nurses and increase the risk that hospitalized patients may develop clinically important complications or worse. If there were plenty of nurses available with the knowledge and skills that hospitals need and hospitals were flush with financial resources, then these concerns could be largely eliminated because hospitals could staff all their nursing units to peak patient levels during every shift of every day. However, such a response is highly unlikely; even if there were enough nurses to staff to peak levels, this would be an inefficient use of nurses and would be prohibitively expensive. In fact, as we discuss in the following section, the changing composition and size of the overall nursing workforce suggest that nurses will become increasingly scarce resource in the years ahead, despite the increased number of nurses returning to the workforce to ride out the current recession.

Nursing Shortages

The most recent hospital nursing shortage began in 1998, when hospitals first reported unfilled positions in ICUs, ORs, and postanesthesia recovery units.[75] The shortage soon spread to medical and surgical units, with the result that in 2001, hospitals reported that the national average vacancy rate for full-time R.N. positions was 13% (vacancy rates greater than 5% are generally considered to indicate shortages). Vacancy rates exceeded 20% in many hospitals, and consequently some hospitals reported closing inpatient units and restricting hours of operation in outpatient and other patient care facilities. Despite increases in R.N. earnings in 2002 and 2003, which helped decrease vacancy rates below double-digit levels, the shortage persisted.

In 2008, however, hospital R.N. employment growth increased dramatically. Because approximately three out of every four R.N.s are married, the recession (which began in December 2007 and has continued well into 2009) resulted in either the real or anticipated loss of employment of the spouses of many R.N.s. Consequently, despite the decrease in R.N. wages in 2007 and 2008, many married R.N.s who had not been employed reentered the workforce, and others who were working on a part-time basis increased their participation to full time. New nursing graduates and nurses from other countries also entered the labor market, resulting in total employment increasing by nearly 250,000 full-time equivalent (FTE) R.N.s.[76] It is anticipated that this unusually large increase in R.N. employment will ease, if not entirely end, the current shortage of nurses in many hospitals. However, relief from the shortage is expected to be temporary, lasting as long as the recession-induced increase in unemployment pressures R.N.s to maintain their increased participation in the workforce.

Changing Workforce Composition

In addition to the persistence of a nursing shortage during most of the current decade, the composition of the nursing workforce has become increasing older. Between 2001 and 2008, total employment of R.N.s increased by an estimated 476,000 FTE R.N.s. During this period, employment of older R.N.s (age 50 to 64 years) increased by an estimated 368,000 FTEs, or 77% of the total increase. With respect to hospitals, 230,000 FTEs, or 59% of the total growth in hospital employment, was accounted for by older R.N.s. In contrast, during these same years net hospital employment growth of middle-aged R.N.s (35–49 years) actually decreased, whereas younger R.N.s (younger than 35 years) supplied 33% of the employment growth in hospitals. In 2006, the average age of the R.N. workforce increased to 43.7 years, and the largest age group was composed of R.N.s in their 40s. The most current projections suggest that the average age will reach 44.5 years in 2012, when R.N.s in their 50s will make up the largest age group in the workforce, numbering roughly 750,000.[77]

The aging of the workforce has mixed implications for hospitals and patient care quality. On the one hand, compared with younger R.N.s, older R.N.s are likely to have greater nursing knowledge, skills, and clinical experience. These characteristics can be important in how effectively nurses prioritize their workload, solve problems, mentor younger nurses, and teach patients about self-care. Older nurses may also be more proficient in detecting patient complications early and knowing how and when to intervene to prevent the complication from worsening and even causing death. (See the discussion about failure to rescue in the preceding section.) On the other hand, compared with younger R.N.s, the bodies of older R.N.s are likely to have greater "wear and tear" resulting from many years of walking, pulling, lifting, stooping, bending, and reaching. Older R.N.s are therefore more susceptible to musculoskeletal injuries and, when injured, require a longer time to recuperate. In fact, a 2008 national survey of R.N.s found that nearly half (45%) reported having musculoskeletal injuries during the previous year.[3] Thus, as the future hospital R.N. workforce is composed of a greater proportion of older R.Ns., the capacity of the nursing workforce to adjust to surges in patient demand is likely to be compromised.

Future Shortages

Because the many R.N.s born during the baby boom generation have not been replaced by younger R.N.s, not only is the average age of the current workforce increasing, but the rate of growth in the supply of R.N.s will decrease as baby boom R.N.s retire during the next decade. Although larger cohorts born in the 1970s and 1980s will prevent the R.N. workforce from decreasing in size, these cohorts are not large enough to add enough R.N.s who will be required to meet the projected demand, which is expected to increase by 2% to 3% per year during the next 20 years. In addition, limited openings in nursing schools and an insufficient number of teachers constrain the number of nurses entering the field.[78] Consequently, a projected shortage of R.N.s is expected to develop by roughly 2015, increase to an estimated 285,000 FTE R.N.s by 2020 (nearly three times larger than any deficit experienced in the United States during the past 50 years), and expand to roughly 500,000 R.N.s by 2025.[75] Importantly, should this projected shortage develop, it will fall on a much older R.N. workforce than did shortages experienced in previous decades.

Given an aging R.N. workforce and projected large shortages developing during the next decade, R.N.s will become increasingly scare resources. At the hospital nursing unit level, the declining physical ability of older R.N.s means that nurses will be less able to accommodate the increased workload brought about by uncontrolled surges in patient demand. As a result, the likelihood that some nurses may not provide needed patient care could increase and, in turn, increase patients' risk of developing complications. Given changes in hospital payment systems based on pay for performance, hospitals' financial health may be negatively affected if nursing shortages lead to an increase in "never

conditions." In addition, because of the expected large future shortage, hospitals that do not exert greater control over patient flow will be at increased risk that nurses will leave for other hospitals that act to smooth or minimize peaks in patient demand, thereby providing their nursing staff with greater predictability and lowering their overall workload.

Controlling Sources of Variability in Patient Census

The overriding goal of this chapter is to increase hospital decision makers' recognition of the numerous negative effects of poorly controlled patient flow on hospital systems of care and the individuals affected by them. As we have described, the effects are complicated and often interconnected and have consequences for patients and hospital staff. Surges in patient demand require managers and nurses to gather, filter, and process large amounts of information and coordinate the actions of many individuals in an effort to prevent systems from faltering. When systems break down, patients are at increased risk of experiencing complications or adverse outcomes during their hospitalization. Although systems do not usually collapse and patients are not harmed, the response of hospital staff who contend with repeated cycles of surges in patient demand come at the cost of staff burnout, stress, and fatigue. These costs are shared with hospitals, which pay for hours of unnecessary overtime, excessive use of temporary staff, and needless and costly replacement of staff who leave to work elsewhere. Unless decision makers share in recognizing these problems, it will be difficult to take effective action to reduce them.

This chapter is also intended to ensure that hospital decision makers recognize that the nursing workforce will be increasingly unable to respond effectively to the problems created by poorly controlled patient flow. The aging of the R.N. workforce means that many R.N.s will be unable to provide the physical effort required by their jobs. In addition, the large shortage projected to develop during the next decade means that hospitals are unlikely to have access to enough R.N.s to respond to the expected growth in patient demand, let alone meet surges in patient demand. The importance of adequate nurse staffing was made clear in recent parallel surveys of physicians and the public that focused on perceptions of medical errors.[79] A little more than half (53%) of physicians and a majority (65%) of the public identified understaffing of nurses in hospitals as very important causes of medical errors. Physicians reported only two approaches as very effective in reducing errors: "requiring hospitals to develop systems to avoid medical errors" (55%) and "increasing the number of hospital nurses" (51%).[80]

As a consequence of high-profile disasters in the United States such as the September 11, 2001, attacks and Hurricane Katrina, efforts have increased to improve large-scale surge management capabilities.[81,82] However, far less effort has been directed at addressing the more insidious threats to safety and quality that arise from frequent surges in patient demand brought about by controllable (and thus preventable) increases in patient admissions. As illustrated in the vignette, surges in unplanned admissions created boundary conditions that forced managers and nurses to make difficult decisions that often involved trade-offs in quality and safety. As surge cycles are repeated and staff repeat their response to adapt to them, compromised care delivery practices can become accepted as customary. Over the longer term, systems designed to protect and maintain care quality and patient safety are undermined. However, by taking control of potentially controllable sources of patient flow, management can reduce the risk that care delivery systems will drift unwittingly into unsafe, low-quality practices.

Taking Control of Patient Flow Management

Subsequent chapters (Chapters 4 and 6–8) describe the actions that management can take to minimize the frequency and magnitude of unnecessary surges in patient demand. Therefore, we bring this chapter to a close by describing some of the benefits that are likely to ripple through a hospital's care delivery systems as a consequence of more assertive patient flow management. At the hospital supervisor level, controlling surges in patient demand can be expected to increase the certainty of staffing levels across units and decrease the overall use of costly temporary nurses. Freed from the conflicts and time involved in finding and allocating staff, supervisors can focus more of their time on improving systems and processes of care and interacting with staff and coworkers. For example, supervisors can develop stronger relationships with community-based providers so that the needs of discharged patients are better matched with community-based resources. Should hospital payments be bundled and extended to include 30 days postdischarge, it is in a hospital's economic interest to decrease readmissions, which are also a source of uncontrolled patient arrival at the ED. Nurse supervisors could also spend more time mentoring nursing unit managers and other nurses so that when patient demand surges and other crises inevitably occur, managers and clinicians can respond more effectively by being able to draw on stronger relationships and more effective communication and by having a better understanding of the strengths and weaknesses of subsystems (for example,

pharmacy, admitting, housekeeping). Closer supervisor involvement with nursing unit mangers and staff can help increase coordination, decrease mistakes and lapses in safety, reduce work-arounds, and help eliminate duplicated efforts, all of which weaken a hospital's clinical and economic performance.

Many of these same benefits also accrue to unit charge nurses. Relieved of the time-consuming and annoying burden of cajoling, exhorting, and persuading reticent or unwilling nurses to work an extra shift to staff peaks in patient demand, charge nurses can instead focus more of their time ensuring that unit-based standards of quality and safety are met and exceeded. Mangers can work more frequently and meaningfully with staff to design and test experiments to improve care systems and focus on the needs of nurses, such as improving the ergonomic environment to help reduce musculoskeletal injuries. Increased efforts to achieve shared clinical and organizational goals can strengthen nurses' commitment to their units, promote staff continuity, and increase retention. Taken together, these outcomes are also likely to lead to improvements in the financial performance of nursing units.

For nurses at the point of care, greater predictability in patient arrival and discharge can be expected to result in fewer interruptions and distractions that will benefit nurses and patients. Greater predictability will help nurses more effectively plan, co-ordinate, deliver and evaluate the outcomes of care activities. At the same time, increased predictability can help decrease the emotional conflicts that many R.N.s confront when they are doing their best to complete all of the care that their patients require but fall short of this goal. Other conflicts that arise when work life intrudes into nurses personal lives can be alleviated, such as the trade-off between overtime and spending that time with family or on other activities. A more stable working environment may also promote a community of practice that fosters collegial relationships among peers and with other individuals with whom nurses interact. Nurses need to know who they can trust to act in predictable ways, particularly during a surge in patient demand or some other crises. Finally, nurses who observe managers taking decisive actions to smooth the peaks in patient demand are more likely to perceive that hospital management cares about them and appreciates the problems and conflicts they face in providing safe patient care. A more supportive management might increase staff commitment to their units and overall loyalty to the hospital and might also encourage nurses to think more about how they can improve patient care and less about finding a different job where the care environment is better.

References

1. Leape L.: Lucian Leape on patient safety in U.S. hospitals. Interview by Peter I. Buerhaus. *J Nurs Scholarsh* 36(4):366–370, 2004.

2. Buerhaus P., et al.: Still making progress to improve the hospital workplace environment? Results from the 2008 National Survey of Registered Nurses. *Nurs Econ,* 27:289–301, Sep./Oct. 2009.

3. Buerhaus P.I., et al.: Impact of the nurse shortage on hospital patient care: Comparative perspectives. *Health Aff (Millwood)* 26:853–852, May–Jun. 2007.

4. Miller A., Xiao Y.: Multi-level strategies to achieve resilience for an organization operating at capacity: A case study at a trauma centre. *Cognition, Technology, & Work* 9(2):51–66, 2007.

5. Miller A., et al.: Clinical communication in a trauma intensive care unit (ICU): A case study. *Proceedings of the Human Factors and Ergonomics Society 52nd Annual Meeting.* 835–839, 2008. http://www.mc.vanderbilt.edu/cprq/publications/Miller%20Clinical%20Comm.pdf (accessed Sep. 11, 2009).

6. Miller A., et al.: Processes and support tools for interhospital neonatal patient transfer: A preliminary study. *Proceedings of the Human Factors and Ergonomics Society 52nd Annual Meeting* 865–869, 2008. http://www.mc.vanderbilt.edu/cprq/publications.html (accessed Sep. 11, 2009).

7. Cook R., Rasmussen J.: "Going solid": A model of system dynamics and consequences for patient safety. *Qual Saf Health Care* 14:130–134, Apr. 2005.

8. Amalberti R., et al.: Violations and migrations in health care: A framework for understanding and management. *Qual Saf Health Care* 15 (Suppl. 1):i66–i71, Dec. 2006

9. Institute of Medicine: *Nursing Staff in Hospitals and Nursing Homes: Is It Adequate?* Washington, DC: National Academy Press, 1996.

10. Institute of Medicine: *To Err Is Human: Building a Safer Health System.* Washington, DC: National Academy Press, 2000.

11. Flood S.D., Diers D.: Nurse staffing, patient outcome and cost. *Nurs Manage* 19:34–43, May 1988.

12. Giraud T., et al.: Iatrogenic complications in adult intensive care units: A prospective two-center study. *Crit Care Med* 21:40–51, Jan. 1993.

13. Archibald L., et al.: Patient density, nurse-to-patient ratio and nosocomial infection risk in a pediatric cardiac intensive care unit. *Pediatr Infect Dis J* 16:1045–1048, Nov. 1997.

14. Amaravadi R., et al.: ICU nurse-to-patient ratio is associated with complications and resource use after esophagectomy. *Intensive Care Med* 26:1857–1862, Dec. 2000.

15. Pronovost P., et al.: Organizational characteristics of intensive care units related to outcomes of abdominal aortic surgery. *JAMA* 281:1310–1317, Apr. 14, 1999.

16. Fridkin S.K., et al.: The role of understaffing in central venous catheter-associated bloodstream infections. *Infect Control Hosp Epidemiol* 17:150–158, Mar. 1996.

17. Cimiotti J.P., et al.: Impact of staffing on bloodstream infections in the neonatal intensive care unit. *Arch Ped Adolesc Med* 160:832–836, Aug. 2006.

18. Needleman J., et al.: Nurse-staffing levels and the quality of care in hospitals. *N Engl J Med* 346:1715–1722, May 30, 2002.

19. Kovner C., Gergen P.: Nurse staffing levels and adverse events following surgery in U.S. hospitals. *Image J Nurs Sch* 30(4):315–321, 1998.

20. Dimick J.B., et al.: Effect of nurse-to-patient ratio in the intensive care unit on pulmonary complications and resource use after hepatectomy. *Am J Crit Care* 10:376–382, Nov. 2001.

21. Unruh, L.: Licensed nurse staffing and adverse events in hospitals. *Med Care* 1:142–152, Jan. 2003.

22. Blegen M.A., Vaughn T.: A multisite study of nurse staffing and patient occurrences. *Nurs Econ* 16:196–203, Jul.–Aug. 1998.

23. Sovie M.D., Jawad A.F.: Hospital restructuring and its impact on outcomes: nursing staff regulations are premature. *J Nurs Adm* 31:588–600, Dec. 2001.

24. Langemo D.K., Anderson J., Volden C.M.: Nursing quality outcome indicators. The North Dakota study. *J Nurs Adm* 32:98–105, Feb. 2002.

25. American Nurses Association (ANA): *Nurse Staffing and Patient Outcomes in the Inpatient Hospital Setting.* Washington, DC: ANA, 2000.

26. Blegen M., Good C., Reed L.: Nurse staffing and patient outcomes. *Nurs Res* 47:43–49, 1998.

27. Aiken L., et al.: Hospital nurse staffing and patient mortality, nurse burnout, and job dissatisfaction. *JAMA* 288:1987–1993, Oct. 23–30, 2002.

28. Scott W., Forrest W., Brown B.: Hospital structure and postoperative mortality and morbidity. In Shortell S., Brown M. (eds.): *Organizational Research in Hospitals.* Chicago: Blue Cross, 1976, pp. 72–89.

29. Hartz A.: Hospital characteristics and mortality rates. *N Engl J Med* 321:1720–1725, Dec. 21, 1989.

30. Aiken L.H., Smith H.L., Lake E.T.: Lower Medicare mortality among a set of hospital known for good nursing care. *Med Care* 32:771–787, Aug. 1994.

31. Schultz M., et al.: The relationship of hospital structural and financial characteristics to mortality and length of stay in acute myocardial infarction patients. *Outcomes Manag Nurs Pract* 2:130–136, Jul.–Sep. 1998.

32. Hamilton K.E., Redshaw M.E., Tarnow-Mordi W.: Nurse staffing in relation to risk-adjusted mortality in neonatal care. *Arch Dis Child Fetal Neonatal Ed* 92:F99–F103, Mar. 2007.

33. Shortell S.M., Hughes, E.F.: The effects of regulation, competition, and ownership on mortality rates among hospital inpatients. *N Engl J Med* 318:1100–1107, Apr. 28, 1988.

34. al-Haider A.S., Wan, T.T.: Modeling organizational determinants of hospital mortality. *Health Serv Res* 26:303–323, Aug. 1991.

35. Shortell S.M., et al.: The performance of intensive care units: Does good management make a difference? *Med Care* 32:508–525, May 1994.

36. Litvak E., et al.: Cost and quality under managed care: Irreconcilable differences? *Am J Manag Care* 6:305–312, Mar. 2000.

37. Litvak E.: Optimizing patient flow by managing its variability. In *Front Office to Front Line: Essential Issues for Health Care Leaders.* Oakbrook Terrace, IL: Joint Commission Resources, 2005, pp. 91–111.

38. Litvak E., et al.: Emergency department diversion: causes and solutions. *Acad Emerg Med* 8:1108–1110, Nov. 2001.

39. Program for Management of Variability in Health Care Delivery: *Improving Patient Flow and Throughput in California Hospitals Operating Room Services.* Prepared for the California HealthCare Foundation, 2007, Chapters 5 and 6. http://www.bu.edu/mvp/Library/CHCF%20Guidance%20document.pdf (accessed Jul. 14, 2009).

40. Litvak E., Cooper A., McManus M.: *Root Cause Analysis of Emergency Department Crowding and Ambulance Diversion in Massachusetts.* Boston: Massachusetts Department of Public Health, Oct. 2002. http://www.mass.gov/Eeohhs2/docs/dph/quality/healthcare/ad_emergency_dept_analysis.pdf (accessed Aug. 25, 2009).

41. McManus M.: *Emergency Department Overcrowding in Massachusetts: Making Room in Our Hospitals.* Massachusetts Health Policy Forum, Jun. 7, 2001.

42. McManus M.L., et al.: Variability in surgical caseload and access to intensive care services. *Anesthesiology* 98:1491–1496, Jun. 2003.

43. Budreau G., et al.: Caregiver–patient ratio: Capturing census and staffing variability. *Nurs Econ* 17:317–324, Nov.–Dec. 1999.

44. Hobgood C., Villani J., Quattlebaum R.: Impact of emergency department volume on registered nurse time at the bedside. *Ann Emerg Med* 46:481–489, Dec. 2005.

45. Ream R.S., et al.: Association of nursing workload and unplanned extubations in a pediatric intensive care unit. *Pediatr Crit Care Med* 8:366–371, Jul. 2007.

46. Robert J., et al.: The influence of the composition of the nursing staff on primary bloodstream infection rates in a surgical intensive care unit. *Infect Control Hosp Epidemiol* 21:12–17, Jan. 2000.

47. Thungjaroenkul P., et al.: Nurse staffing and cost of care in adult intensive care units in a university hospital in Thailand. *Nurs Health Sci* 10:31–36, Mar. 2008.

48. Haley R.W., Bregman D.A.: The role of understaffing and overcrowding in recurrent outbreaks of staphylococcal infection in a neonatal special-care unit. *J Infect Dis* 145:875–885, Jun. 1982.

49. Haley R.W., et al.: Eradication of endemic methicillin-resistant *Staphylococcus aureus* infections from a neonatal intensive care unit. *J Infect Dis* 171:614–624, Mar. 1995.

50. Harbarth S., et al.: Outbreak of *Enterobacter cloacae* related to understaffing, overcrowding, and poor hygiene practices. *Infect Control Hosp Epidemiol* 20:598–603, Sep. 1999.

51. Hugonnet S., Chevrolet J.C., Pittet D.: The effect of workload on infection risk in critically ill patients. *Crit Care Med* 35:76–81, Jan. 2007.

52. Hugonnet S., Uckay I., Pittet D.: Staffing level: A determinant of late-onset ventilator-associated pneumonia. *Crit Care* 11(4):R80, 2007.

53. Upenieks V., et al.: Assessing nursing staffing ratios: Variability in workload

intensity. *Policy Polit Nurs Pract* 8:7–19, Feb. 2007.

54. Dancer S.J., et al.: MRSA acquisition in an intensive care unit. *Am J Infect Control* 34:10–17, Feb. 2006.

55. Halwani M., et al.: Cross-transmission of nosocomial pathogens in an adult intensive care unit: incidence and risk factors. *J Hosp Infect* 63:39–46, May 2006.

56. Tarnow-Mordi W.O., et al.: Hospital mortality in relation to staff workload: A 4-year study in an adult intensive-care unit. *The Lancet* 356:185–189, Jul. 15, 2000.

57. Tucker J., UK Neonatal Staffing Study Group: Patient volume, staffing, and workload in relation to risk-adjusted outcomes in a random stratified sample of UK neonatal intensive care units: a prospective evaluation. *Lancet* 359:99–107, Jan. 12, 2002.

58. Arnow P., et al.: Control of methicillin-resistant *Staphylococcus aureus* in a burn unit: Role of nurse staffing. *J Trauma* 22:954–959, Nov. 1982.

59. Blatnik J., Lesnicar G.: Propagation of methicillin-resistant *Staphylococcus aureus* due to the overloading of medical nurses in intensive care units. *J Hosp Infect* 63:162–166, Jun. 2006.

60. Farrington M., et al.: Effects on nursing workload of different methicillin-resistant *Staphylococcus aureus* (MRSA) control strategies. *J Hosp Infect* 46:118–122, Oct. 2000.

61. Grundmann H., et al.: Risk factors for the transmission of methicillin-resistant *Staphylococcus aureus* in an adult intensive care unit: Fitting a model to the data. *J Infect Dis* 185:481–488, Feb. 15, 2002.

62. Dorsey G., et al.: A heterogeneous outbreak of *Enterobacter cloacae* and *Serratia marcescens* infections in a surgical intensive care unit. *Infect Control Hosp Epidemiol* 21:465–469, Jul. 2000.

63. Mayhall C.G., et al.: *Enterobacter cloacae* septicemia in a burn center: Epidemiology and control of an outbreak. *J Infect Dis* 139:166–171, Feb. 1979.

64. Stegenga J., Bell E., Matlow A.: The role of nurse understaffing in nosocomial viral gastrointestinal infections on a general pediatrics ward. *Infect Control Hosp Epidemiol* 23:133–136, Mar. 2002.

65. Evans W.N., Kim B.: Patient outcomes when hospitals experience a surge in admissions. *J Health Econ* 25:365–388, Mar. 2006.

66. Kalisch B.J., Landstrom G., Williams R.A.: Missed nursing care: Errors of omission. *Nurs Outlook* 57:3–9, Jan.–Feb. 2009.

67. Karmel H.K., et al.: Time to ambulation after hip fracture surgery: Relation to

hospitalization outcomes. *J Gerontol A Biol Sci Med Sci* 58:1042–1045, Nov. 2003.

68. Rasmussen H.H., et al.: Prevalence of patients at nutritional risk in Danish hospitals. *Clin Nutr* 23:1009–1015, Oct. 2004.

69. Mundy L.M., Leet T.L.: Early mobilization of patients hospitalized with community-acquired pneumonia. *Chest* 124:883–889, Sep. 2003.

70. Munin M.C., et al.: Early inpatient rehabilitation after elective hip and knee arthroplasty. *JAMA* 279:847–852, Mar. 18, 1998.

71. Whitney J.D., Parkman S.: The effects of early postoperative physical activity on tissue oxygen and wound healing. *Biol Res for Nurs* 6:79–89, Oct. 2004.

72. Price P., Fowlow B.: Research-based practice: Early ambulation for PTCA patients. *Can J Cardiovasc Nurs* 5(1):23–25, 1994.

73. Yohannes A.M., Connolly M.J.: Early mobilization with walking aids following hospital admission with acute exacerbation of chronic obstructive pulmonary disease. *Clin Rehabil* 17:465–471, Aug. 2003.

74. Pedroja A.T.: The tipping point: The relationship between volume and patient harm. *Am J Med Qual*, 23:336–341, Sep.–Oct. 2008.

75. Buerhaus P., Staiger D.O., Auerbach D.: *The Future of the Nursing Workforce in the United States: Data, Trends and Implications.* Sudbury, MA: Jones & Bartlett, Inc., 2009.

76. Buerhaus P.I., Auerbach D.I., Staiger D.O.: The recent surge in nurse employment: Causes and implications. *Health Aff (Millwood)* 28:w657–w658, Jul.–Aug. 2009.

77. Buerhaus P.I.: Current and future state of the US nursing workforce. *JAMA* 300:2422–2424, Nov. 26, 2008.

78. American Association of Colleges of Nursing: *Nursing Faculty Shortage Fact Sheet,* Jun. 2009. http://www.aacn.nche.edu/Media/FactSheets/Faculty Shortage.htm (accessed Aug. 25, 2009).

79. Blendon R.J., et al.: Views of practicing physicians and the public on medical errors. *N Engl J Med* 347:1933–1940, Dec. 12, 2002.

80. Altman D., Clancy C., Blendon R.: Improving patient safety—Five years after the IOM report. *N Engl J Med* 351:2041–2043, Nov. 11, 2004.

81. Rudowitz R., Rowland D., Shartzer A.: Health care in New Orleans before and after Hurricane Katrina. *Health Aff (Millwood)* 25:w393–406, Sept.–Oct. 2006.

82. Felland L.E., et al.: Developing health system surge capacity: Community efforts in jeopardy. *Res Briefs* 5:1–8, Jun. 2008.

Chapter 3

Assessment of Patient Flow

Brad Prenney, M.S., M.P.A.

A hospitalwide assessment of patient flow can provide a foundation on which an effective strategy can be developed and implemented to meet The Joint Commission's Leadership standard for managing patient flow, Standard LD.04.03.11: "Leaders develop and implement plans to identify and mitigate impediments to efficient patient flow throughout the hospital."[1] An assessment can put a hospital in a better position to (1) understand where patient flow problems exist, their causes, interrelationships, and impact, and (2) formulate and implement an effective, comprehensive strategy for improvement, which is what the Leadership standard calls for. Although some patient flow improvements can be undertaken in its absence, a full-scale hospitalwide patient flow assessment is generally necessary to support an integrated and comprehensive effort to improve patient flow across major service areas of a hospital.

This chapter provides guidance on integrating suggested strategies for patient flow assessment for implementing the Leadership standard.[2] The approach for carrying out a patient flow assessment centers on patient demand variability, the underlying cause of the systemic patient flow problems experienced by hospitals. The American Hospital Association's Hospitals in Pursuit of Excellence program has adopted the following as one of its six principles: "Manage organizational variability. Some variables, such as scheduling of elective surgery, can be smoothed out to achieve more even patient flow."[3] Accordingly, a comprehensive effort to evaluate hospital patient flow should begin by assessing organizational variability in patient demand. The demand variability approach derives from operations management (OM) principles and practices. OM application is particularly suited to the hospital care environment because of the many different patient flow pathways that exist. In addition, the characteristics of these pathways differ, the pathways frequently have many steps and are interconnected, and the pathways share resources, often creating the potential for competition.

Finally, the chapter, with its focus on performing a hospitalwide assessment of patient flow (system assessment), does not address assessment of patient flow across care delivery systems (intersystem assessment; for example, primary care to acute care to postacute care) or within individual service areas (service-level assessment). Approaches for analyzing patient flow across a multidimensional framework have been presented by others.[4]

Variability as a Key to Assessment

Patient flow is a key to understanding a hospital's operational efficiency. In an efficient hospital care delivery system, each patient served is provided the right care at the right time and in the right place. To achieve that goal during each patient encounter, the necessary resources (that is, capacity) must be available to serve that patient demand for services. In an ideal patient flow system, resources in the form of an appropriate bed, nurse, test, or procedure are immediately available whenever a patient requires that service. When more resources are available than are needed to serve patient demand, waste results; excess capacity exists in a system where services cannot be inventoried. When those resources are lacking, the system is stressed and patient flow problems result. Waits, delays, rejections, cancellations, and misplacement, all of which represent problems related to timely access to appropriate care, are manifestations of patient flow problems and operational inefficiencies. *Variability in patient demand for services (flow variability) is the primary cause of these problems.*[5]

Demand for service is generally driven either by patient arrival patterns (for example, patients arrive to the emergency department [ED] seeking services); time of completion of the previous care delivery step(s) (for example, radiology examination before treatment); and/or scheduling practices (for example, when surgeons book operating room [OR] time to perform their cases). These patterns can be highly variable. Hospitals often attempt to deal with these variable demand flows by altering capacity to bring it in line with presenting demand.[6] However, because these demand patterns are often random, transient, and/or unpredictable, adjusting capacity to meet variable demand is rarely successful in a practical, real-time sense and as an overall strategy. Approaching the problem from the demand side of the equation requires that patient demand variability either be eliminated or managed in such a way as to minimize those instances when demand and capacity are out of sync.

Within this context, assessment of patient flow attempts to identify where patient demand variability exists, to understand its causes and its impact, and to use that knowledge as the basis for developing strategies to manage it.

The approach has the following objectives, generally carried out in sequence:
  1. Identify patient demand variability.
  2. Characterize the variability.
  3. Identify the source of the variability.
  4. Establish and quantify its impact.
  5. Determine how to manage or eliminate it.
The assessment attempts to provide answers to the first four objectives so that recommendations can be formulated that determine how best to manage or eliminate variability.

Must you undertake a hospitalwide patient flow assessment before attempting to improve patient flow in one or more service areas? The answer is *no*. Patient flow problems affecting specific service areas can be addressed with success without undertaking a comprehensive patient flow assessment. Redesign of the OR, for example, to eliminate competition for OR resources between scheduled and unscheduled surgical demand will improve patient flow for surgical patients, especially those who present to the ED for treatment. Carried out properly, the OR redesign effort would involve some level of assessment of existing patient flow problems in the OR. Although a specific improvement initiative such as this may have a beneficial outcome on hospitalwide patient flow, the benefit may be limited if major sources of patient demand variability remain unidentified and unaddressed, especially those originating in other service areas, such as electively scheduled surgical admissions.

Should a particular hospital undertake a hospitalwide patient flow assessment before trying to undertake patient flow improvement? The answer is *maybe*. Answering this question comes down to a matter of judgment and strategy, as reflected in the following questions:.
  ■ Are key stakeholders in agreement about what needs to be done to address the patient flow problem(s)?
  ■ Do they have to be in order to successfully address the problem?
  ■ Is the expected impact of the improvement effort on patient flow clearly understood?
  ■ Are there other patient flow problems that exist that will not be impacted by the improvement effort?
  ■ How important are these?
  ■ Does the improvement represent the most optimal utilization of time and resources available to address patient flow problems in the hospital?

Whether a hospital should perform a formal hospitalwide patient flow assessment before (or even concurrently with) undertaking patient flow improvement(s) is a question that is best left to each hospital.

There are other process improvement approaches and methodologies, most notably Lean and Six Sigma,[7] that can and have been used to assess and improve patient flow in the hospital environment. Process mapping of patient flow pathways can be useful in identifying care delivery steps that are duplicative or can be eliminated, resulting in streamlining of the care delivery process and a reduction in service time.[8] Identifying process defects and setting acceptable limits for process outcomes can also have benefits in improving service times and patient flow.[9] The assessment methodology described in this chapter, although focusing on the system-level impact of patient demand variability, does include a certain level of service-level process assessment. Can you undertake service- or process-level assessment in parallel with undertaking a hospitalwide assessment of patient flow assessment? *Yes*, that too is possible. However, that decision should be based on practical considerations, including resource and time requirements.

Getting Started

Defining the Scope of the Assessment

Defining the scope of the effort is generally the first major challenge in performing a patient flow assessment. There are innumerable patient flow pathways in a hospital. An assessment cannot realistically examine all of them or even most of them. The goal is to identify the major patient flow problems affecting the hospital system and to use the assessment as the basis for developing and implementing an effective patient flow management strategy. Two considerations in defining what patient flow pathways to assess are (1) major patient demand flows and (2) flow streams that cross service areas and/or involve shared resources.

In most hospitals, the two major portals for entry are through the emergency department (ED) and elective admissions.[10] Transfers can also represent a significant source of patients, especially for tertiary care facilities. Surgical services are often the major source of elective admissions but not always. In some cases, a particular service may be experiencing patient flow and other operational problems, and you will decide to assess this area because it represents a priority or problem area, although it is not a major patient flow pathway. For example, the number of patients undergoing cardiac catheterization may pale in comparison to the number of ED admissions or surgical operations performed. However, because catheterization laboratory patients compete with ED admissions for telemetry beds, one may decide to include this service as part of the assessment.

The importance of particular hospital services is not simply defined by their volume. There could be other reasons why a particular patient flow stream is important to consider. For example, where particular patient flow streams compete with other streams for shared services (beds, OR resources, ancillary services, ICU), one will often uncover patient flow bottlenecks and consequent problems of waits, delays, and rejections because of the competition for shared resources. Sometimes the sharing (or competition for resources) can occur among a patient flow stream that is largely separate from other hospital services and patients. For example, obstetrical patients generally do not compete for services with ED or surgical patients. Maternity beds are typically used solely for these patients. Obstetrical patients normally have their own ORs or their own OR blocks and staff and recovery areas. Nevertheless, patient flow problems in the obstetrical service can be a major area of concern for the hospital. Often the problem stems from the fact that within the obstetrical service there can be competing patient flows, possibly reflecting different arrival patterns. Women giving birth naturally can be expected to arrive at the hospital in a random pattern, while women who are being induced or giving birth by cesarean section are more often scheduled. Poor scheduling practices can result in these flows competing for OR space, beds, staff, and so on, resulting in patient flow problems unrelated to what is going on in other areas of the hospital.[11]

In attempting to define the scope of the assessment, it is important to consider what hospital services are used by various patient flow streams. Outpatients, by definition, are not admitted to the hospital, so you would not expect them to compete for inpatient beds, unless they have been admitted for less than 24 hours of observation. However, they do use other services, many of which are shared with inpatients (for example, OR resources, postanesthesia care unit [PACU] beds, ancillary services). With the exception of ED patients (treated and discharged), most outpatients are scheduled. Scheduling practices can create patient flow bottlenecks. Also, while awaiting discharge, outpatients can sometimes be held in beds and recovery areas that are used by other patient flow streams, including inpatients.

The service areas to be assessed are not just those that correspond to major patient flow streams entering the hospital (for example, ED patients, surgical patients, outpatients, obstetrical patients). Ancillary services are often important to assess because they provide services to multiple patient flow streams. For example, radiology, pharmacy, and laboratory services are used by a wide variety of specialties and patient populations. Radiology procedures, especially computerized tomography and ultrasound, may be accessed by inpatients and outpatients, leading to ED backlogs. Demand for these services is rarely internally generated but rather is determined by external demand (*see* Figure 3-1, page 32). As a result, these services can have patient flow and operational problems imposed on them by demand patterns dictated elsewhere. In addition, inefficiencies associated with the provision of ancillary services can create delays or extended service times that can impact patient flow.

Mapping the various patient flow streams in the hospital can be helpful in identifying the pathways and patient flows that you want to include in the assessment. A schematic representation is

Figure 3-1. Arrived Clinic Visits That Needed X-ray by Date, Nonholiday Weekdays, September 1–30

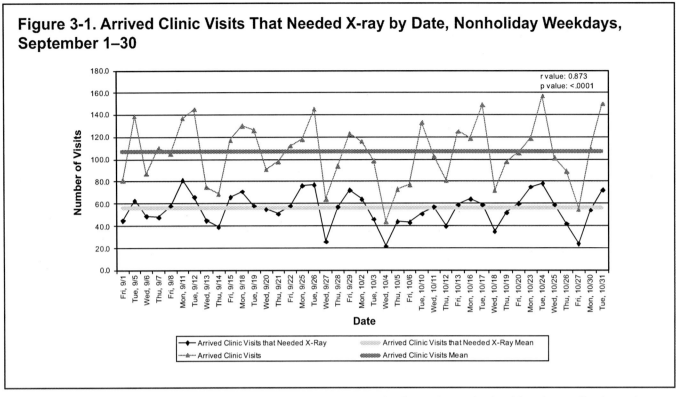

Ancillary services, such as radiology, as reflected in this figure, can be subject to patient flow and operational problems imposed by demand patterns dictated elsewhere.

also useful in identifying the relative importance of various services and pathways that are shared (*see* Figure 3-2, page 33). Where quantitative information on volume is unavailable, being able to establish the relative size of these pathways should be sufficient in determining where major flow pathways exist. Developing an input–output model of movement of patients to and from hospital inpatient units can be helpful in defining the scope of the assessment.[8]

Decisions should be made deliberatively regarding the scope and level of service-level process analysis that will be performed as part of the assessment. Process mapping of the major service areas that will be assessed can be useful in understanding how care is delivered and the sequence of steps followed in that service area.[12] Whether each of those individual process steps should be examined for bottlenecks and inefficiencies should be established at the outset while considering the limits in available time and resources for the assessment.

It can be easy to get lost in the forest of interconnected flows, questions, and data associated with the assessment and lose sight of its goals. Defining the scope of and successfully carrying out an assessment are inherently challenging because of the complexity and diversity of hospital care delivery. Not only are there myriad patient flow pathways, but patient flow problems can occur both as a result of system-level bottlenecks (in which a constraint affects

another service area, such as the lack of ICU beds causing surgical patients to be held in the PACU) and by inefficiency and capacity/demand imbalance internal to the service area (for example, delays in the ED caused by an insufficient number of triage staff).

In attempting to establish the scope of the assessment, it is generally worthwhile to seek input from hospital representatives as well. If a patient flow committee has been established, it may be a good starting point for identifying service areas that are experiencing patient flow problems.

As the analytical process unfolds, you may find that one set of analyses leads to a set of new questions and issues to be explored. Multiple bottlenecks may be uncovered. The sources of some of the bottlenecks and their impacts, as well as the interrelationships among the bottlenecks, might not be clear. In trying to digest and make sense of the analyses and apparent findings, keep the overall goal of the assessment—to identify system-level sources of patient flow problems—clearly in mind. Inefficiencies within service areas may be contributing factors to patient flow problems, but they are unlikely to be root causes. Targeting service areas and delivery steps where resources are shared will also focus the findings. Those areas that represent a source of a major patient flow stream or have a significant potential impact on other service areas, upstream or downstream, are areas where you will want to focus the findings.

Figure 3-2. Schematic Representation of Patient Flows

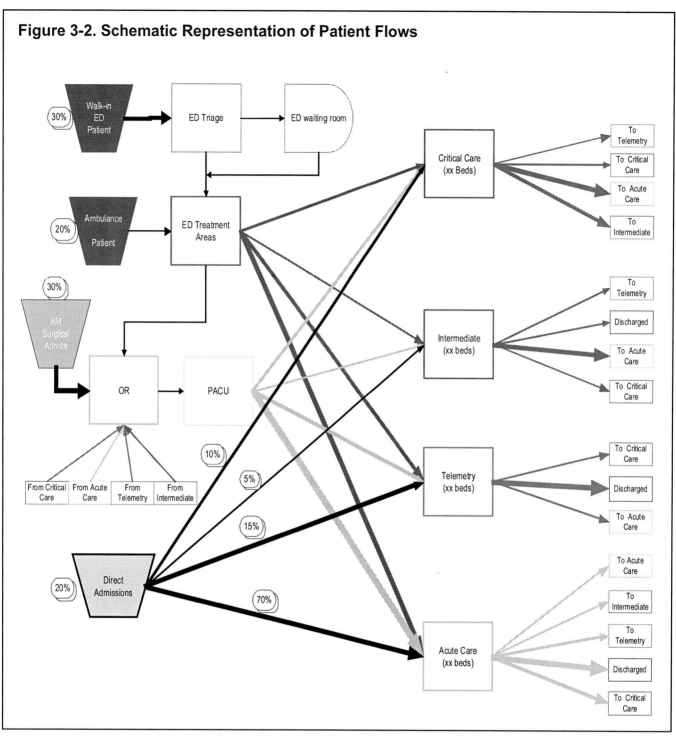

A schematic representation of patient flow is useful in identifying the relative importance of various shared services and pathways. For example, in this sample schematic representation, different flows compete to varying degrees for each category of inpatient beds (for example, *70% of direct admissions go to acute care beds). ED, emergency department; AM, morning; OR, operating room; PACU, postanesthesia care unit. Used with permission.*

Early on in the assessment, especially prior to staff interviews and discussions, hospital leadership should decide in what form and in what manner the assessment findings and recommendations will be presented to hospital staff. Participants in the assessment phase will naturally want to know how the information they provide (for example, during the interviews) will be used and whether the hospital will share the findings and recommendations when the assessment is completed. These are important questions to consider beforehand.

Organizational Support

There should be leadership support for carrying out a patient flow assessment. This support should be obtained and announced early on in the process and presented in the context of a larger effort to improve operational efficiency and patient flow. Clinical and administrative leaders, both at the service and hospital levels, should buy into the assessment process and understand—and preferably agree—that the findings and recommendations that flow from the assessment will form the basis for implementing improvements. Key individuals are more likely to participate in the process if they know how it relates to the overall goal.

Many hospitals have created patient flow committees that have broad hospital representation and provide a forum and mechanism for sharing and addressing patient flow problems. Such a committee or another such multidisciplinary team can be very helpful in identifying patient flow problems and in assisting in coordinating the assessment and follow-up improvement initiatives. Project management resources are normally required to effectively carry out the assessment. Whether dedicated, full-time project management is necessary depends on the scope of the assessment and the role and responsibilities expected of project staff in the implementation stage to follow. Someone who is currently leading a hospitalwide patient flow committee may be a good candidate for overall project management because he or she would be familiar with operational and patient flow issues and would have worked with key service representatives.

Data collection and analysis can be the most challenging and time-consuming aspect of the assessment effort. Good candidates to lead the data collection and analysis portion of the project would be individuals who have experience with using hospital data for decision support, reporting, and performance improvement and who are familiar with hospital operations. Direct care staff also have an important role in guiding the analyses and in interpreting findings. For example, an ED nurse may be in a good position to confirm that the time a care delivery step is recorded in the information technology (IT) system is an accurate indicator of the time of an event.

Understanding Terminology and Operations

To properly assess patient flow, it is important to understand how patient flow streams arrive and move through the system and what resources they utilize and when. Understanding the terminology used by hospital staff, clinicians, administrators, and support personnel not only in their day-to-day interaction but in the record-keeping and data systems that they maintain is vital to an assessment. A hospital employee charged with leading an assessment might think that terminology is not an issue for her because

she is generally familiar with the clinical, operational, and administrative terms used by staff. However, staff discussions may well prove otherwise. For example, whether or not patient arrivals, procedures, and so on are scheduled or unscheduled, or even inpatient or outpatient, is important in assessing and characterizing patient demand variability. The information, as documented by staff or available data systems, rarely falls neatly into mutually exclusive categories. In the OR, unscheduled cases might consist not only of cases that are clinically emergent or urgent, semiurgent, or semielective but also of cases that are "added on" or "worked in" to the schedule on the day of or the day before surgery. Cases performed in the catheterization laboratory or in obstetrics may have different terms applied to them with regard to scheduling and clinical urgency.

Further categorization should be performed with regard to whether the case requires hospital inpatient services on leaving the PACU. Same-day surgery and other categories may be employed. It is important to determine what postoperative resources are used by each of these categories. Various cross-tabulations of these categories should be carried out so that their relationships are clearly understood (*see* Table 3-1, page 35).

Digging below the surface of terms, labels, and categories may uncover information necessary to adequately understand patient flow in the hospital. For example, outpatients or same-day surgery patients may in fact occupy inpatient beds, even if temporarily, while they await discharge. Even though those patient are not admitted or do not stay overnight, they compete with inpatients for the same beds. Therefore, assuming that all outpatients are discharged after diagnostic/treatment procedures and do not compete for shared inpatient resources would be erroneous. In addition, understanding scheduling practices and identifying whether arrival patterns are patient or provider driven is critical in understanding the type of variability that may be affecting patient flow in the system and, ultimately, taking appropriate steps to eliminate or optimally manage it.

Data Needs

In a patient flow assessment, data analyses establish findings that will form the basis for the development of recommendations to address patient flow problems. Management and clinical staff observations and opinions on patient flow issues and problems are useful in helping to establish the scope of the assessment, in identifying operational areas of concern, and in determining what data are needed to carry out the assessment. However, they generally should not be relied on as the basis for establishing assessment findings. If you are unable to establish that the problem exists

Table 3-1. Case Types and Patient Categories

CASE TYPE	AM	IN	OP	PDC	SDC	SDC*	Missing Patient Categories	Grand Total
	1							1
Added	3	57			7	10	7	84
Emergency	1	63			6	7	17	94
Scheduled	256	96		9	600	188	37	1186
	1	3	1		2	2		9
Grand Total	262	219	1	9	615	207	61	1374

AM, morning; IN, inpatient; OP, outpatient; PDC, pediatric day care; SDC, surgical day care; SDC*, < 24 hours. Used with permission.

analytically, then you should appropriately qualify any findings based on subjective information and think very carefully before making recommendations on how to address the perceived problem.

Time Elements

Data that indicate the time that events took place are critical to carrying out an assessment. Why? Given the multiple interconnected steps in the hospital care delivery process, an ideal patient flow system would be represented by patients moving immediately, without delay, to the next, appropriate step in the care delivery pathway once service is completed. Under these ideal conditions, a patient flow assessment would hardly be needed but could be easily carried out if one were able to track the time that the patient arrived and departed at each of the care steps. Conditions in real life, however, are not ideal, and no hospital can claim to have eliminated patient flow problems.

In the real world, a patient flow problem can manifest itself as delay (or wait), extended service time, cancellation, service rejection, or suboptimal service. Using hospital data to determine whether one or more of these consequences exist is the analytical basis for establishing that a patient flow problem exists. This is the logical prelude to determining its cause and formulating a recommendation to improve the situation.

Time elements are needed to establish whether patients wait for a service or experience delays during the receipt of the service. Time elements that indicate when a service began and when it ended for each patient normally form the basis for carrying out the assessment. With these data, one can track patient flow movement in the hospital.

Another important role of time elements is to determine a potential flow bottleneck. A simple rule of doing so is as follows:

> If waiting time, T_w, to get to a particular unit is noticeably greater than the boarding* time, T_b (waiting time till the downstream unit is available), in this unit, then this unit is a potential bottleneck. If, however, $T_b > T_w$, the bottleneck is likely to be in one of the downstream units.

(*A common definition of boarding is "holding an admitted patient beyond two hours."[13])

However, patient movement alone does not necessarily inform you as to whether there were waits and delays. It is important, if at all possible, to distinguish through the data analysis between when a patient arrives or departs a service area and when he or she should have arrived or departed on the basis of clinical condition or time of the care provider's decision to move to the next care delivery step. That difference in time (between when a patient actually arrived and departed and when he or she should have arrived and departed) represents the manifestation of patient flow problems that result in delays, waits, and extended service times.

Data Files

Existing hospital data contained in administrative and service-level databases are normally sufficient to carry out an assessment. In particular, the admission/discharge/transfer (A/D/T) data system, maintained by all hospitals, can be a rich source of information for assessing patient flow into and out of the hospital, as well as between hospital units. In most hospital assessments, the data elements and information available are less than ideal, and some data elements may not be available. For example, hospitals might not capture the time that a patient was ready to move on to the next step in the care delivery process or when a clinical decision was made that could represent an adequate proxy. Being able to distinguish between the clinically driven length of stay (LOS) during a step in the care delivery process and that portion of the actual service LOS caused by delay would be ideal. However, many times those data elements are not available. Actual LOS will often suffice in an effort to identify patient flow problems. Delays and waits will be manifested in varying LOS for particular patients or during specific time periods. The collection of prospective data can be time-consuming and expensive and should be avoided because it is generally not required to carry out an assessment.

Databases maintained by various services (for example, ED, OR/PACU, radiology) are also needed to carry out an assessment. These databases generally contain data elements necessary to characterize and examine the patient flow streams through the various care pathways. They allow one to determine time of entry and departure from the service, delays experienced, the characteristics of the patients, and when and what tests and procedures were provided and by whom. They also contain information (for example, medical record number, account number) that allows one to link various databases so that patients' progression and destination can be determined.

Before carrying out the analyses, it is important to review the data sets for quality and completeness. Cleaning of the data can be a time-consuming process, but it is critical for the analyses and related findings to be considered and presented with reliability and confidence. The upfront investment is worthwhile. As a rule, patient flow analyses of data files should be carried out only after a data file has undergone a quality review. The initial quality review should identify the data elements and values contained in the file, determine whether the file is complete, and determine whether the range of values for individual data elements fall into a reasonable or expected range. Data files from a particular service area should be reviewed with an eye to establishing consistency and identifying errors in the data. For example, calculated LOS should always be a positive number, departure times should be later than arrival times, and OR and PACU numbers should be relatively consistent. Certain data elements have a direct relationship that can be examined to evaluate the quality of the data as, for example:

Average Case Duration × Case Volume = Total Surgical Minutes or

Departure Time —

Arrival Time = LOS

Data quality review should be performed on an ongoing basis because a set of analyses result in further questions to be explored. A thoughtful and deliberate determination of the specific question to be answered or, say, table or figure to be created before undertaking the analysis builds the necessary focus and discipline into an analytical effort where it is easy to get lost in the forest of analyses.

Use of Information Technology and Other Advancements

The use of IT and related technological advancements to assess and monitor patient flow has been highly recommended in recent years.[14] Bed status systems, electronic dashboards, and so on have been added to the arsenal of management tools to track, in real-time, the status of resources and movement of patients through the hospital care delivery system. The use of radio frequency identification (RFID) tags to track patients, as well as equipment, has also received much attention in the assessment of hospital patient flow. However, it is important to keep in mind these systems' limitations. Although they may be able to track patient movement, they do not necessarily provide information regarding when a patient should have or was clinically ready to move to the next step in the care delivery process. Also, using information collected principally for real-time tracking of patient movement to analyze patient flow across systems may require a certain level of IT/programming support to create usable data files for a patient flow assessment.

In formulating what data are needed to carry out the assessment, it is important to keep in mind the longer-term goal of being able to evaluate patient flow on an ongoing basis and to be able to assess the impact of patient flow improvement initiatives. For those critical data elements that are either not collected or cannot be readily used in existing form, this initial stage of the assessment can bring attention to the need to revise IT/data systems so that these data elements can be routinely captured and used for ongoing assessment purposes and to evaluate the impact of improvement initiatives.

Other Information Needs

Conducting the patient flow assessment not only provides the basis for formulating recommendations and strategies for improving flow but also serves to build consensus and support for change. An effective assessment can be extremely valuable to hospital administrators and clinicians in addressing contrasting views of the causes of operational problems and overcoming resistance to change.

Patient flow problems manifest themselves in various ways. In addition to bottlenecks, which, as already stated, can result in delays, waits, and extended service times, there are other consequences, including cancellation of service, rejection of patient demand, and suboptimal care. Ambulance diversion is a prime example of the rejection of patient demand. When the ED becomes overcrowded (normally because of the inability to move admitted patients to the floors), a hospital may go on ambulance diversion as a way of temporarily lowering demand for ED and inpatient services. External or internal policies and practices may affect how a hospital responds to a patient flow bottleneck. For example, in states in the United States where ambulance diversion is not allowed, hospitals do not have the option of diverting ambulance traffic. In these states, the assessment is carried out with the knowledge that rejection of demand is unlikely to be a consequence of patient flow problems in the ED.

Internal policies also influence how a hospital responds to patient flow bottlenecks. One major consequence of patient flow bottlenecks is *patient misplacement.*[15] When a patient is ready to be admitted from the ED or leave the PACU, for example, the unit most appropriate for that patient might not have a bed available. As explained in Chapter 1, one option would be to hold, or "board," the patient in the ED or PACU until a preferred bed becomes available on the unit. However, boarding the patient may result in backups in the sending unit (for example, ED) or upstream in the OR. The hospital might decide to send the patient to a different unit where a bed is available, even though the bed in that unit may be less appropriate from a clinical care standpoint. Establishing that this type of consequence is associated with patient flow problems is as important as establishing that delays exist, and it can be valuable in linking patient flow problems to diminished quality of care. Therefore, it is important that the assessment include review of formal admission criteria established by the hospital for placement of ED, surgical, and other types of patients. This review can also be valuable in designing ways to better manage patient demand. For example, community-based physicians frequently want their patients who come through the ED or as direct admissions to be placed in monitored beds (telemetry units) even though they do not meet admission criteria. This additional demand on telemetry beds can be one major reason why existing capacity is inadequate to meet demand (for example, from the catheterization laboratory as well as the ED). Establishing this practice as part of the assessment can be the basis for recommending increased compliance with existing admission criteria as a way of effectively managing patient demand. Similarly, it is important to take into account discharge criteria that have been established by the hospital. Extended service times (LOS) on some units may be a result of the inability (for example, difficulty placing patients in nursing homes or postacute care rehab beds) or unwillingness (for example, nursing staff delaying discharge until shift change or limiting new admissions) to discharge patients when they are ready to leave the unit.

Other hospital policies and practices may also affect patient flow. For example, delay in transporting patients from one step in the care delivery process to the next affects patient flow. However, a policy that requires or results in a nurse transporting the patient when doing so is not clinically necessary may well delay admission

of new patients to the unit. The policies and practices that might affect patient flow or be affected by patient flow problems should be evaluated as part of the assessment, preferably early, when the scope of the assessment is being determined. Interviews with staff from major service areas that will be assessed are often an opportune time to raise policy and practice issues before formulating the list of data elements needed to perform analyses.

Impact of Previous Patient Flow Efforts

As part of the assessment, it is frequently beneficial to evaluate and understand the steps that might have been previously taken to address patient flow problems. This information will identify actions that may have mitigated or even exacerbated the problem or altered its impact or manifestation. For example, a common reaction to ED overcrowding or the inability to get OR cases performed is to expand capacity, under the assumption that the source of the problem resides where the consequences are being felt. When the bottleneck resides downstream (for example, inpatient or PACU beds in short supply), expanding capacity upstream from the constraint can add further pressure on the bottleneck without improving flow. In addition to adding capacity, hospitals will sometimes create "buffer" units to offload some of the demand (for example, chest pain unit in the ED, holding area for discharged patients). Although this may ameliorate the patient flow problems, it comes at a cost.

Even the basic care delivery model established for the inpatient units may have undergone alteration in response to patient flow problems. For example, telemetry beds may have become scattered throughout the hospital over time because of the inability to routinely and in a timely manner admit patients to the established telemetry unit. Technology investments and process improvement initiatives may also have been instituted in response to patient flow problems. As the assessment proceeds to its conclusion, putting these previous efforts into the proper cost–benefit perspective will put the hospital in a better position of charting future actions.

Analyses

General Considerations

Although most hospitals are "open" or operate 24 hours a day, 7 days week, the reality is that the level of activity and types of services offered changes considerably on the weekends and holidays as compared with weekdays. The activity in most hospitals falls off over the weekend and on holidays. Typically, very little if any elective surgery occurs over the weekend, and volume can drop considerably on a holiday. Corresponding PACU activity can decline as well because census and availability of ancillary services and staffing may be reduced. This should be confirmed with some basic analyses examining volume of activity for seven days a week across the various service areas being assessed. This is important to consider because a different level of activity will affect demand for services. This has bearing on the focus of the assessment—that is, on identifying, understanding, and describing variability in patient demand for services. Therefore, including weekends and holidays in the basic analyses may amplify and introduce variability that should be considered structural and distinct from variability that one intends to either eliminate or manage. The change in level of activity might not be found for certain services, such as the ED, where the volume of visits can be relatively constant across the seven-day workweek. In general, however, analyses should focus on nonholiday weekdays, although it might be beneficial to analyze data for the entire week to explore potential incremental hospital capacities/throughput under a seven-day operations scenario.

Variability in patient demand for services presents itself as change from one particular time period to another, which can be expressed in terms of arrivals, departures, number of visits, admission rate, volume of procedures, and so on. Analysis to uncover variability, therefore, focuses heavily on examining activities or events by time parameters such as date, day of week (DOW), and hour of day. There are various ways of measuring and expressing the magnitude of the variability found, including the following:

- The percentage difference from the mean of peaks and valleys of a pattern can help reflect the range of variability.

- The calculation of standardized residuals (sum of the absolute difference between each "event" and the mean) can be used to compare the relative size of variability (and each contribution) among two or more patterns being analyzed.

- The coefficient of variation allows one to take into account different means among patterns of variability being examined.

Once variability is identified and its magnitude examined, characterizing the type of variability is the next step. Analyses can be very helpful in establishing what is driving the event or the service activity. A pattern that shows average demand varying across specific days of the workweek is not uncommon. For example, a hospital's finding that the average number of surgical cases arriving to the PACU from the OR is highest on Thursday might conform to staff perceptions and provide support for the view that staffing levels can be adjusted to reflect this higher volume on that day. The assumption might be that the Thursday volume of PACU arrivals is routinely high relative to other days of the week, and it is predictable. However, analyses that examine PACU arrivals across all Thursdays in the time period being studied would suggest otherwise (*see* Figure 3-3, right). Typically, you find that volume levels vary considerably across Thursdays. Some

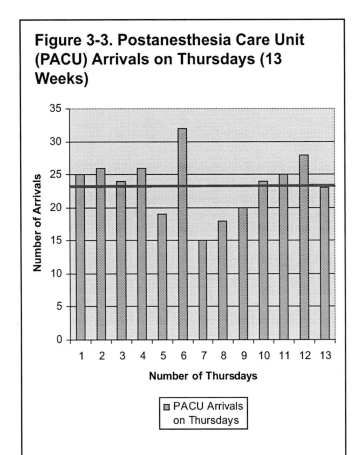

Figure 3-3. Postanesthesia Care Unit (PACU) Arrivals on Thursdays (13 Weeks)

It is often found in day-of-week analyses that volume levels vary considerably across a given day of the week. The horizontal line represents the mean.

Thursdays could see patient volume close to the average, but often it is not. This helps point out the limitation of certain analyses (such as DOW) and indicates that variability can be both nonrandom and unpredictable. Assuming, therefore, that because a particular workday has on average a greater or lesser volume of demand than other weekdays does not mean that setting staffing levels at a higher or lower level to match that average demand will eliminate instances of misalignment between capacity and demand. In fact, every Thursday's volume could depart from the overall average.

Judgments regarding the efficiency of a hospital unit or service are often based on impressions, perceptions, and selected experiences of hospital clinicians, managers, and staff. There is a natural tendency to recall the periods when demand peaked rather than the valleys in demand and to view those periods of stress as typical and reflective of the unit's normal operations. Certain types of analyses can debunk those impressions and put into proper perspective the effects of variable demand. Figure 3-4 (page 39) displays the volume of catheterization laboratory procedures for each weekday for a three-month study period. Although some days

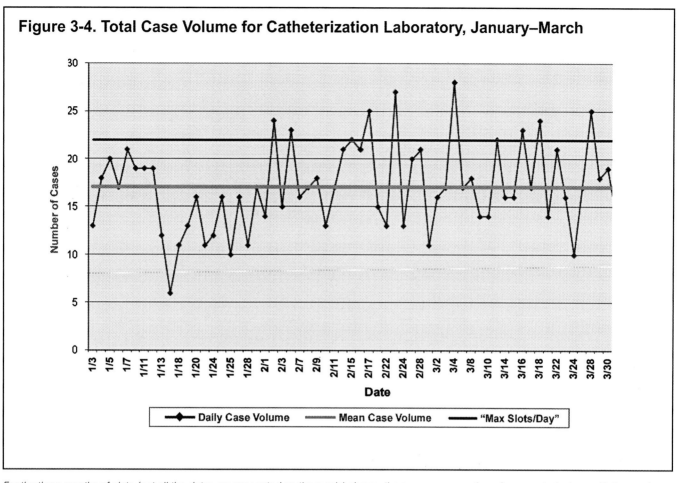

Figure 3-4. Total Case Volume for Catheterization Laboratory, January–March

For the three months of data (not all the dates are presented on the x axis) shown, the average case volume is presented, along with the maximum number of catheterization laboratory slots allotted per day. SR, standardized residuals (as defined on page 38), is 21%, and the utilization rate is 78%, at an average of 44 slots per day. Note that despite relatively low utilization, there are frequently days when the catheterization laboratory is overwhelmed and days when capacity lies idle.

have an average volume of procedures, on many days volume is at or above the maximum level of slots, resulting in stress and overtime. On other days, volume is far below the allotted slots. Yet overall utilization of catheterization laboratory resources is less than optimal, at 78%, especially for procedures that are by and large scheduled and for which procedure length is fairly predictable. Utilization should be at least 90%, so that the analyses indicate a system that is paradoxically routinely stressed yet underutilized.

Before examining patient flow in and across service areas, it is normally worthwhile to assess patient flow and demand variability across the hospital as a whole. This can be done by examining overall patient flow into (admissions) and out of (discharges) the hospital, along with overall census by the fundamental time metrics of date, DOW, and hour of day. The three hospital parameters have a fundamental relationship—that is, arrival rate and LOS determine discharge rate—but might be influenced by a variety of other factors. For example, arrivals (admissions) could be largely a function of admitted patients arriving randomly to the

ED, along with scheduled surgical and medical admissions, whereas discharges may be affected by the timeliness and availability of postacute care destinations, along with service times and delays encountered during the hospital stay (for example, home transport, nursing home placement). Admission and discharge patterns are also influenced by hospital policies and practices (for example, workups and admission orders written toward the end of shift, discharge rounding taking place in the late morning). Examining these patterns by time parameters can reveal when there are stresses on the system (arrivals and discharges peak or when beds are fully occupied) and, conversely, when demand is lowest and resources may lie idle. The hour-of-day patterns may be particularly important in identifying whether the admission and discharge processes are "desynchronized"—and are thereby affecting patient flow (*see* Figure 3-5, page 40).

Admission Analyses

A first step in analyzing data on patient flow is to examine admissions to the hospital by the standard time parameters date, DOW,

Figure 3-5. Average Admissions Versus Discharges, by Hour, All Days February 1–April 30

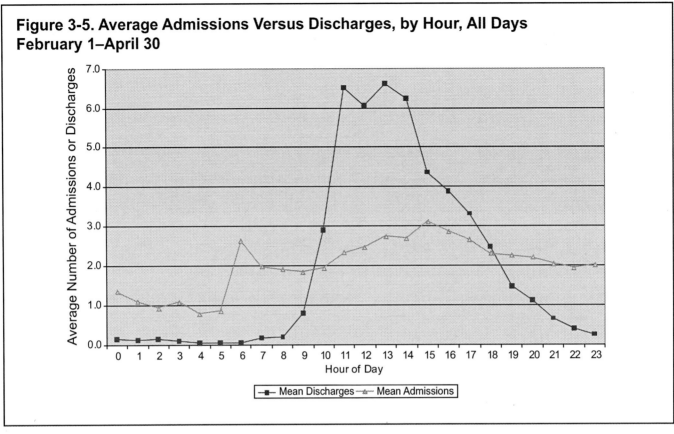

Excluding early-morning surgical admissions, admissions peak only after midday discharges.

and hour of day. This will establish the overall flow of patients into the hospital and the extent of variability in arrivals during nonholiday weekdays for these time parameters.

Patients arrive to the hospital through various portals of entry—for example through the ED, as direct admissions, elective admissions, or transfers. It is useful to both identify and quantify the volume of each of these flows and again establish the extent of variability over time. It should be established whether each of these categories of admissions represent scheduled and/or unscheduled admissions. Where the arrival stream is unscheduled, you will want to determine whether the pattern is random. Unscheduled admissions, especially through the ED, may have an artificial variability component (not entirely random arrivals), for example, reflecting community-based physicians' referral of patients to the ED for admission on one or more particular week days. This can be tested by determining if the arrival distribution follows a Poisson distribution (*see* Chapter 5). Statistical tests of significance can also be applied to the DOW analyses to determine whether mean volume of arrivals varies significantly across the workdays.

When comparing the extent of variability among scheduled and unscheduled admissions, it may be useful to calculate and compare standardized residuals among the two groups to determine the

individual contribution of each to hospitalwide variability in admissions (*see* Figure 3-6, page 41, and Figure 3-7, page 41).

The analyses should include examining admission patterns by hour of day. This should be done for total admissions as well as for each type of flow. Admission groups may have distinctly different hour-of-day distributions (*see* Figure 3-8, page 42). Comparison of hour-of-day arrivals for scheduled and unscheduled admissions should also be performed. These are unlikely to be uniform, and when compared later with discharge patterns, will allow one to examine synchronization between the admission and discharge processes in the hospital overall. *Where there is lack of synchronization, one is likely to find bottlenecks or underutilized capacity.* These basic hospitalwide admission analyses will enable you to identify the major flows and portals of admission into the hospital, which will be useful in determining the scope of the assessment.

Discharges

An initial step in the analysis of patient flow with respect to discharge issues is to look at the overall pattern of discharges by date, DOW, and hour of day to establish the presence of variability (*see* Figure 3-9, page 42). Variability can be based on a number of

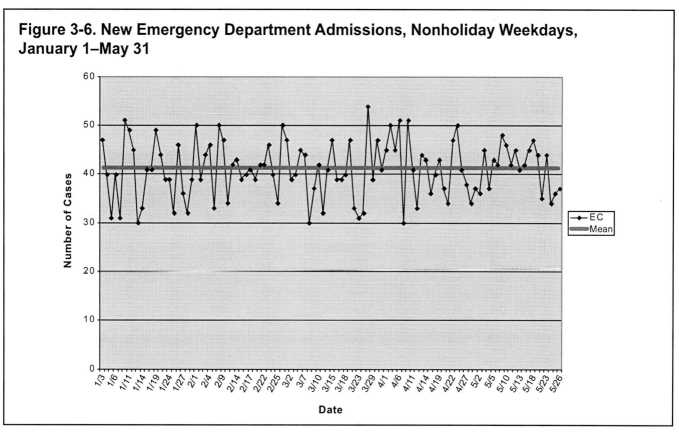

Figure 3-6. New Emergency Department Admissions, Nonholiday Weekdays, January 1–May 31

The number of new ED admissions is shown for nonholiday weekdays during a five-month period. The extent of day-to-day variability in admissions from the ED is relatively modest (SR [standardized residuals], 12%, when compared with new operating room admissions) (see Figure 3-7).

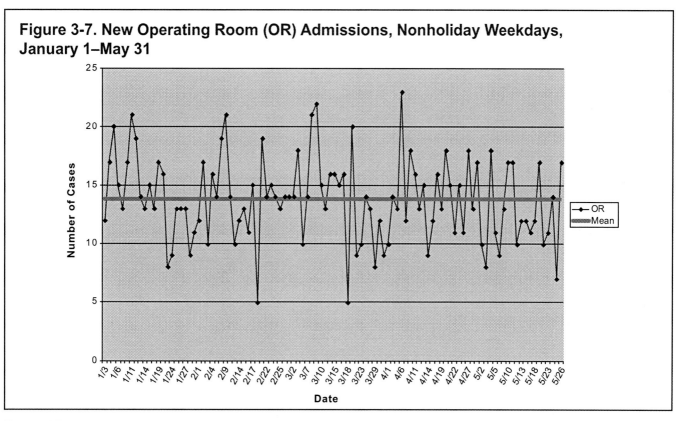

Figure 3-7. New Operating Room (OR) Admissions, Nonholiday Weekdays, January 1–May 31

The new OR admissions, as cited in Figure 3-6, are shown.

Figure 3-8. New Hospital Admissions by Source and Hour, Nonholiday Weekdays, January 1–May 28

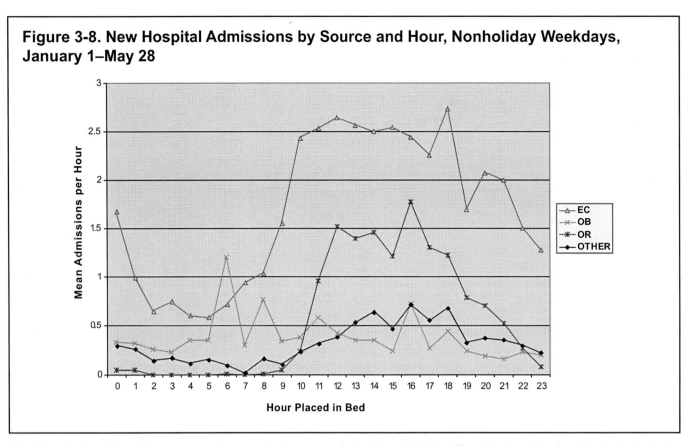

Admissions by hour follow distinct patterns when examined by source of admissions. Note the different hourly pattern for obstetrical patients who have dedicated beds and that of the other groups that share (and compete for) inpatient beds. EC, emergency center; OB, obstetrics; OR, operating room.

Figure 3-9. Discharges by Day of Week, Nonholiday Weekdays Only

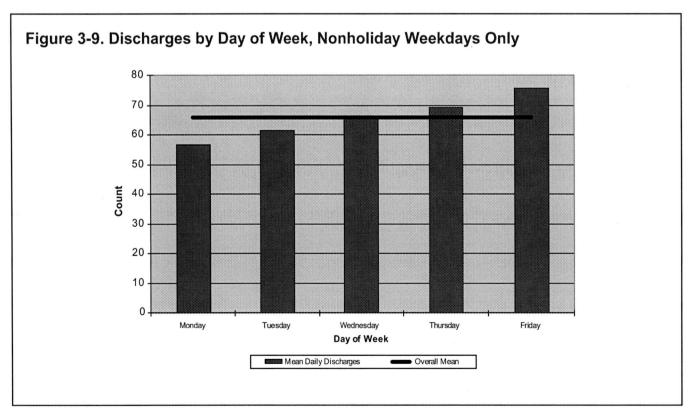

The data (covering a three-month period) indicate that average discharges for nonholiday weekdays increase from Monday to Friday. The horizontal line represents the mean.

factors, some of which are hospitalwide in their effects, others of which affect only some groups of patients. For example, hourly discharge patterns may reflect when physicians round on their patients and write discharge orders. Because services may be significantly reduced on weekends and/or physicians prefer not to round on those days, discharges may increase substantially toward the end of the workweek. Discharge patterns for particular groups of patients may be affected by the availability of postacute care services; for example, skilled nursing facilities may admit patients only at certain hours of the day.

It is useful to correlate overall and specific discharge patterns with corresponding admission patterns, especially on an hour-of-day basis, because it may indicate a lack of synchronization between movement into and out of the hospital or particular units.

Transfers into or out of the hospital, which require resources, compete for beds, and so on, need to be accounted for. For some hospitals (tertiary or quaternary care facilities), transfers may represent a significant volume of admissions and discharges. It may be useful to analyze this group separately because there might be policies or practices that are resulting in variability in patient demand for hospital services. For example, a consortium of

hospitals might accept patients from community hospitals who need specialized care, and the pattern of admissions of these transfers may be dictated by specific policies that rotate these admissions among the participating referral centers.

Census

Analyzing overall hospital census by date, DOW, and hour of day will reveal the extent of variability in overall hospital occupancy or in the occupancy of major groups of inpatient units. It is important to distinguish between licensed and staffed beds. Normally, we focus on staffed beds, which is a better indicator of the use of existing nursing resources. DOW analyses provide an overall view of when the hospital normally fills up or empties out. If census is measured more than one time each day, it would be worthwhile to run the analyses at several times, depending on when the information is collected. Hospitals are likely to experience variable census throughout the day, and if this is the case, it should be documented (*see* Figure 3-10, below).

Examining census at the same hour for one weekday during the study period can be useful in demonstrating unpredictability of the census, probably indicating that artificial variability may lie behind the overall occupancy pattern (*see* Figure 3-11, page 44).

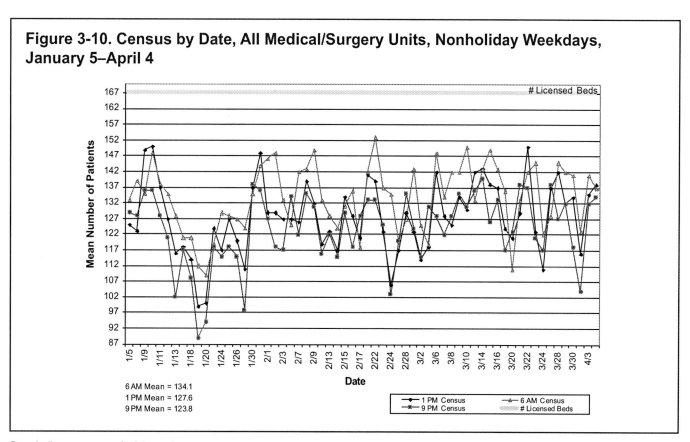

Figure 3-10. Census by Date, All Medical/Surgery Units, Nonholiday Weekdays, January 5–April 4

6 AM Mean = 134.1
1 PM Mean = 127.6
9 PM Mean = 123.8

Data indicate a mean of 134.1 patients at 6 A.M. (06:00), 127.6 patients at 1 P.M. (13:00), and 123.8 at 9 P.M. (21:00), demonstrating that average overall census in these units varies depending on the time of day.

Figure 3-11. Noon Census on Medical/Surgical Units Combined

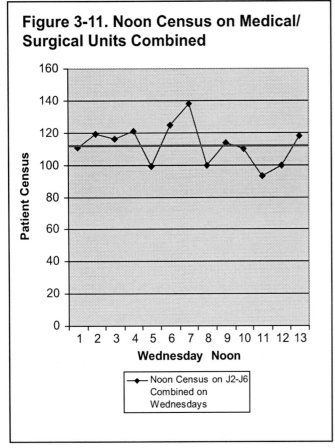

Wednesday Noon

Noon Census on J2–J6 Combined on Wednesdays

The census varies considerably across Wednesdays and frequently differs from the overall average. The horizontal line represents the mean.

Emergency Department

A hospital's ED is typically a major focus of a hospitalwide patient flow assessment for the following three reasons:

1. A high proportion of patients seeking hospital services arrive through the ED.

2. ED patients often compete for resources with patients admitted through other portals (especially elective admissions).

3. Patient flow problems can affect ED in a major way, with important consequences.

The assessment should examine and characterize flow into the ED. Mode of arrival (for example, walk-ins, ambulance transport), which could be affected by overcrowding conditions, as when a hospital goes on ambulance diversion, should be examined. Examining the proportion of ED visits that arrive by ambulance may uncover times when arrivals by this transport mode decline for particular days and/or hours of the day, indicating times of rejected demand due to overcrowding. In some cases, hospitals may collect information on when they go on ambulance

diversion. Volume of arrivals should be analyzed by date, DOW, and hour of day. These analyses should also be performed for each group of ED visits that do and do not result in admission. Because admitted patients require inpatient services, they can be differentially affected by overcrowding conditions and inpatient patient flow bottlenecks. The rate of admissions (proportion of ED visits resulting in admission) can be expected to be relatively constant over most weekdays (Mondays may be the exception if admissions decline on weekends). Different rates may indicate that admission decisions can be affected by overcrowding conditions, especially for patients for whom the decision to admit is not clinically clear-cut. Outpatients are often treated on a separate track (for example, fast track), generally have a shorter and less involved length of stay in the ED, and are often less subject to patient flow problems originating in the ED and inpatient services.

Generally, patients arriving to the ED are not scheduled. Their arrival time is determined largely by when a patient becomes injured or sick and seeks hospital care. Statistical tests can be applied to an arrival pattern (for example, by date of arrival) to determine if it follows a random pattern (or Poisson distribution). However, there can be a nonrandom or artificial variability component to the pattern of ED visits or visits that result in admission. For example, community-based physicians may hold office hours on particular days, and the flow of referrals to the ED for workup and admission may be higher on some days or during certain times of the day. *This is important to establish because artificial variability can potentially be eliminated or reduced, thereby smoothing the flow of ED admissions.* Random, or natural, variability must be managed, and the application of queuing theory to do so generally requires that the arrival pattern be random.

The analyses should attempt to establish whether ED overcrowding conditions exist and whether consequences of patient flow bottlenecks, either in the ED or in other service areas, are affecting ED patients. Examining ED census data can identify times when ED beds are full. Patient flow problems affecting ED patients can be manifested as waits, rejections, service disruption, misplacement, and boarding (in beds or hallways).

Boarding. Many hospitals collect boarding data, which should be used for the analyses, if available. Analyzing boarding statistics (for example, number of boarders, time of boarding) by standard time parameters can uncover patterns indicative of patient flow bottlenecks (*see* Figure 3-12, page 45). Analyses regarding whether certain types of admitted ED patients are being boarded and their intended and actual inpatient destinations should help pinpoint the source of the bottleneck (*see* Figure 3-13, page 46). If boarding time is unavailable, then analysis of ED LOS may be sufficient to pinpoint times of bottlenecks and suggest their sources. Keep

Figure 3-12. Average Wait Time for Bed by Hour of Day, ED Admissions, All Days February 1–April 30

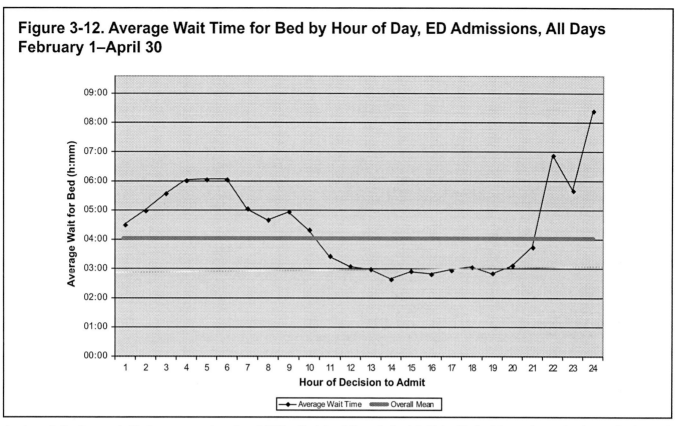

As shown in the figure, admitted emergency department (ED) patients' wait times for beds is highest in the late evening and early morning hours. 1, 1 A.M.; 24, midnight. The horizontal line represents the mean.

in mind that LOS may vary among different types of ED admitted patients because of clinically based diagnostic and treatment requirements. For that reason, LOS is a less reliable statistic for examining boarding. Correlating wait times in the ED with other hospital metrics, such as census, may establish further evidence that patient flow problems occur when the hospital is full or beds are unavailable on particular units.

In conjunction with these analyses, observations of clinical staff should be considered with regard to operational and patient flow problems in ED, diagnostic, admission, and workup processes and in inpatient services. These observations may indicate the need for related types of analyses. Keep in mind that hospitals may have taken certain steps to mitigate or reduce boarding of patients, such as the establishment of a buffer unit to offload patients during times of overcrowding or a policy that allows patients to be boarded in hallways of inpatient floors. These efforts should be analyzed because they assume their own costs and benefits as alternatives to the boarding of ED patients.

Ambulance Diversion. Ambulance diversion—the most common form of rejection resulting from ED overcrowding—represents an attempt to lower demand for services when capacity is insufficient to serve that demand. In addition to establishing

when it occurs, the assessment should also examine the consequences of lost demand. Data are often available to at least estimate, if not precisely determine, what volume of patients and contribution margin may have been lost because of the need to go on diversion. Whenever quality of care consequences can be attributed to ambulance diversion (or any of the other consequences and actions taken to address ED overcrowding), they should be noted and included in the assessment.

Disruption of Service. Another consequence of ED overcrowding due to patient flow problems is disruption of service. This generally takes the form of patients who leave without being seen (LWBS) or leave against medical advice (AMA), usually because of long waits for service. This should be explored and, if data are available, appropriate analyses should be performed to determine the time and frequency of occurrence (*see* Figure 3-14, page 47). Comparisons can be made with diversion and boarding statistics to determine whether common patterns emerge. The financial impact can also be analyzed.

Patient Misplacement. Patient misplacement is another consequence of patient flow problems. If the ED has admission criteria for certain subgroups of patients (for example, chest pain patients sent to telemetry), it may be worthwhile to determine

Figure 3-13. Mean Emergency Department (ED) Length of Stay (LOS) by Type of Unit on First Admission, Nonholiday Weekends, January–May

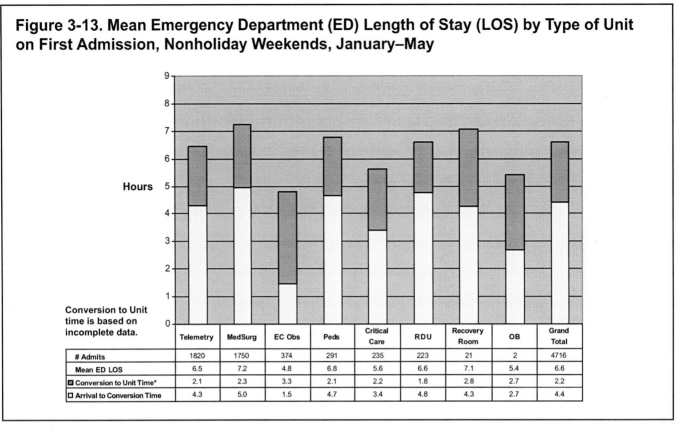

	Telemetry	MedSurg	EC Obs	Peds	Critical Care	RDU	Recovery Room	OB	Grand Total
# Admits	1820	1750	374	291	235	223	21	2	4716
Mean ED LOS	6.5	7.2	4.8	6.8	5.6	6.6	7.1	5.4	6.6
Conversion to Unit Time*	2.1	2.3	3.3	2.1	2.2	1.8	2.8	2.7	2.2
Arrival to Conversion Time	4.3	5.0	1.5	4.7	3.4	4.8	4.3	2.7	4.4

The figure allows one to examine differences in service and "hold" times for patients group with different destinations from the ED, which can help identify downstream patient flow bottlenecks. "Conversion time" (to unit), which indicates the admission decision time, is based on incomplete data.

whether patients routinely go to those preferred units. When they do not, it may indicate where the source of an inpatient bottleneck lies. Times (DOW or hour of day) when patients are sent to other-than-preferred units may coincide with increased demand for beds in the preferred unit from elective flows (for example, catheterization laboratory patients competing with ED patients for beds in the telemetry unit). Also, knowing when misplacement occurs can be useful in identifying periods of severe stress and patient flow problems.

Summary. The importance of documenting the impact that patient flow problems have had on ED operations cannot be overstated. By establishing these impacts, the hospital is in a stronger position of making the case for change and establishing the relationship between scheduling and policy practices in other service areas and their effect on the ED.

In assessing patient flow in the ED, it is worth examining processes internal to the ED that may affect flow. Areas of focus can be identified through interviews with ED and other hospital staff. For example, inefficiencies might be found in the processing of patients through the ED (registration or triage delays), in the receipt of timely diagnostic testing (radiology backups), or in the

admission process itself (hospitalist delays in writing admission orders or delays in workups). Mapping process steps can be useful in identifying possible internal bottlenecks. Examining service times, if available, for these individual processes can uncover steps that experience inappropriately long service times. These analyses, coupled with staff observations, may be sufficient to identify internal bottlenecks. The decision of how extensively to analyze individual ED processes should be made keeping in mind the time, resource, and data constraints, along with the overall goal of the assessment.

Operating Room Services

For the following reasons, the OR service is by far the most important service to examine as part of a hospitalwide patient flow assessment:

1. Surgery represents one of the major sources of flow into the hospital, usually accounting for 30%–40% of admissions.
2. The OR is a major source of revenue for the hospital.
3. The OR shares resources (for example, floor beds, ICU, ancillary services) with a number of other flows, in particular medical patients, many of whom arrive through the ED through transfers or as direct admissions.
4. Surgical patients compete for OR resources.

Figure 3-14. Mean Number of Patients Who Left Without Being Seen (LWBS), Sunday–Saturday

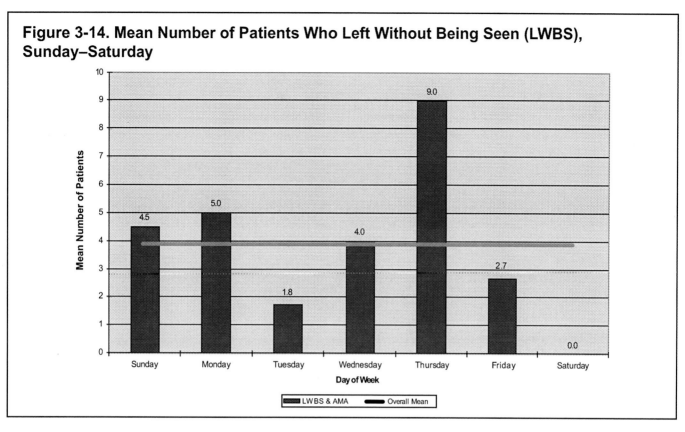

The mean numbers of patients who left without being seen or before disposition for a five-month period, including weekends, are shown. AMA, leave against medical advice.

5. The OR both affects patient flow and is affected by patient flow problems in other areas.

6. The perioperative process is complex, with various sub-services (preop, OR, recovery, inpatient care) involved.

Basic information should be collected about perioperative services as the first step in the assessment process. The following information can be useful in providing background to and context for the assessment analyses that will be performed:

- Preoperative steps and resources
- Number of ORs and prime-time hours
- How turnover time is defined and measured
- Surgical subspecialties and surgeons
- How OR time is allocated and the rules regarding use and release of allocated time
- Types of cases performed (for example, outpatients/same-day surgeries, inpatients) and what resources they use and share
- Backlog of and wait times for different types of surgical cases
- Relationship of surgeons and anesthesiologists with regard to the hospital
- Number and type of PACU beds
- Scheduling practices
- Terms and nomenclature for cases and activities

Fundamental to an assessment of the OR are analyses that examine how and when different types of surgical cases utilize OR resources. These analyses allow one to determine the type, nature, and extent of variability of patient demand for surgical and downstream services. Determining whether a surgical case is scheduled is an important first step in the analytical process.

The terms used to describe how cases arrive to the OR should be examined closely because it is unlikely that, operationally, staff and available data systems neatly categorize cases as either scheduled or unscheduled—or outpatient and inpatient. There may be other categories, for example, such as "add-ons" and/or "work-ins," which reflect cases that get added to the OR schedule the day of or the day before surgery. Surgeries should also be categorized with regard to clinical urgency for performing the surgery. Beyond elective and emergent surgical cases, some cases may be classified as urgent, semiurgent, or semielective. Further categorization should be performed with regard to whether the case requires hospital inpatient services upon leaving the PACU. Same-day surgery and other categories may be employed. It is important to determine what postoperative resources are used by each of these groups. Various cross-tabulations of these categories should be carried out so that their relationships are clearly understood (Table 3-1).

Once these analyses are carried out, one can begin to analyze surgical case activity for the various subgroupings by the basic time parameters. Comparison of case volume by date, DOW, and hour of day for various categories can identify the extent of patient demand variability for surgical cases that are scheduled or arrive randomly to the OR (*see* Figure 3-15, below). A major objective of this part of the OR assessment is to determine the extent of variability associated with the way surgical cases are scheduled. Other types of OR metrics besides case volume should be examined. Because surgical cases differ with regard to the time it takes to perform the procedure, examination of total surgical minutes can be informative in relating variability to use of OR time (*see* Figure 3-16, page 49).

An assessment of patient flow in the OR can often be extended to include an evaluation of the efficiency of day-of-surgery activities and the ability to accurately allocate OR time for cases that vary in procedure length. Analyses of start times, scheduled case duration, and OR turnover time (TOT) are all valuable in assessing how day-of-surgery efficiency affects patient flow (*see* Figure 3-17, page 49, and Figure 3-18, page 50).

The pre- and postoperative care delivery steps are important to examine as part of assessing patient flow through the perioperative process. Delays and cancellations may be caused by inefficiencies in the various processes that occur before the patient enters the OR. Preoperative patient flow problems may be identified by staff during the interviews. Cancellations and delays in start times might indicate inefficiencies and delays in obtaining consent, performing histories and physicals, conducting preoperative testing, and so on.

Surgical activity in the OR directly affects the workload of the PACU, which is generally the next immediate step in the care delivery process for patients coming out of surgery. As part of the assessment, you will want to identify variability not only in the OR but the PACU. Examining volume of arrivals to the PACU by date, DOW, and hour of day will uncover variability in demand that can be compared to OR volume to determine whether similar patterns emerge as expected.

The inability to move patients efficiently through the OR and PACU can be a result of OR case scheduling practices that create peaks in demand for OR time and PACU beds. Patients are often held in the OR until a PACU bed becomes available. This can be established by examining PACU census and OR hold times by hour of day.

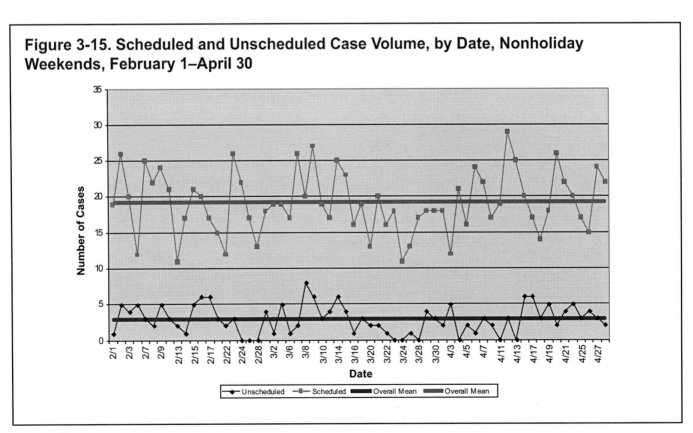

Figure 3-15. Scheduled and Unscheduled Case Volume, by Date, Nonholiday Weekends, February 1–April 30

The data indicate that case volume is much more variable across weekdays for scheduled than for unscheduled cases, a pattern typically seen in patient flow assessments.

Figure 3-16. Total Operating Room (OR) Actual Minutes, Nonholiday Weekdays, February 1–April 30

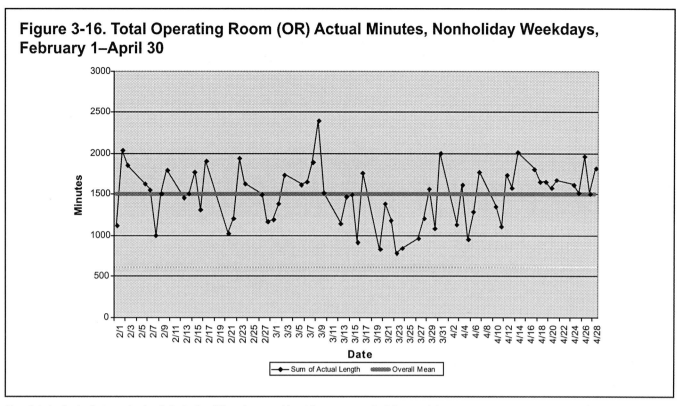

The data indicate that surgical activity in the OR varies considerably across nonholiday weekdays.

Figure 3-17. Distribution of Operating Room (OR) Case Lengths, Nonholiday Weekdays

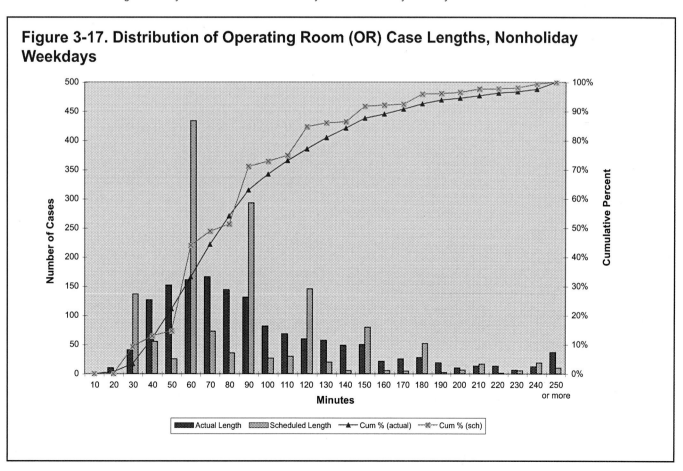

The data indicate that scheduled case length follows an overall cumulative pattern similar to actual case length. Note the effect of scheduling cases at defined hourly intervals. Cum, cumulative.

Figure 3-18. Distribution of Operating Room (OR) Case Start Times, Nonholiday Weekdays

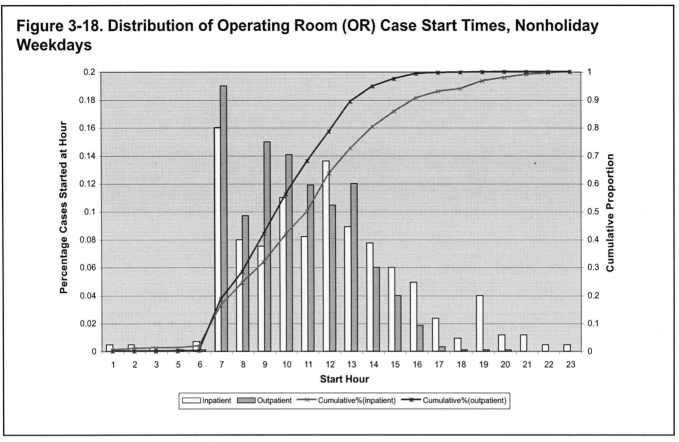

The data indicate that inpatient cases tend to start later in the day.

Patient flow problems in the PACU can also be due to downstream bottlenecks in the inpatient units where patients leaving the PACU are sent. When beds are unavailable, patients can be held in the PACU until a bed becomes available. This can be the cause of backups in the OR; the lack of beds on the floor means that patients are unable to move out of the PACU, and, in turn, surgical patients are being held in the OR while waiting for PACU beds.

Determining when PACU holds occur is important in tying the problem to its source. Some hospitals routinely collect information on PACU hold times. More often, the only data available pertain to overall LOS in the PACU, which generally includes both the clinically necessary time a patient stays in the PACU and wait (hold) time. Although the former time element is preferable in examining PACU delays, LOS can often be a reasonable proxy for investigating when delays occur and the possible source of the delays, as long as surgical case mix is taken into account. Comparing census in downstream units with PACU census and/or average LOS by DOW and hour of day can often establish a correlation between PACU holds and lack of available beds.

Surgical subspecialties often prefer to send their patients to

specific inpatient units from the PACU because of nursing skills, unit care capability, proximity, and so on. When beds in the preferred unit are not available at the time a surgical patient is ready to leave the PACU, the patients may be held in the PACU or sent to a unit other than the one preferred. This should be examined as part of the assessment because misplacement and/or boarding may have quality of care and patient flow consequences. Examining when misplacement and boarding occur will provide an indication of when patient flow bottlenecks arise in downstream units, which may reflect, for example, different flow streams competing for the same beds (for example, ICU).

Other Procedure Services

The patient flow assessment should be applied to other service areas, such as the catheterization and electrophysiology laboratories, obstetrics, and interventional radiology, in which operative and treatment procedures are performed. These areas, too, have internal processes and interrelationships with other service areas in which patient flow is affected by scheduling practices, clinical urgency, shared resources, and downstream needs (*see* Figure 3-19, page 51, and Figure 3-20, page 52).

Figure 3-19. Distribution of Scheduled and Unscheduled Cases in Labor and Delivery, by Hour of Day, Nonholiday Weekdays, February 1–April 30

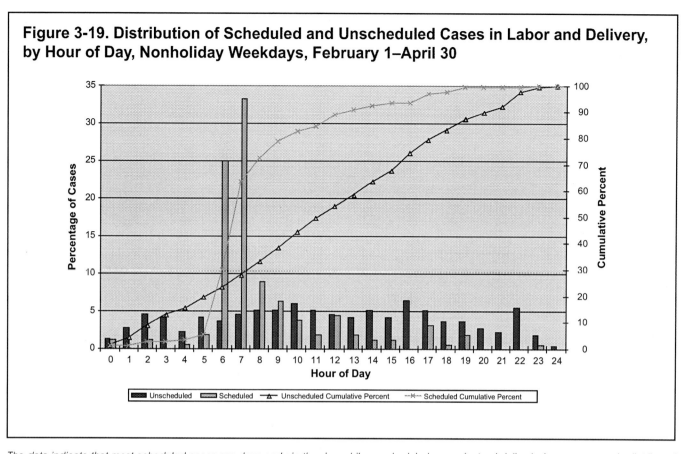

The data indicate that most scheduled cases are done early in the day, while unscheduled cases (natural deliveries) are more evenly distributed across the day, as would be expected.

Date, DOW, and hour-of-day analyses will reveal variability in patient demand. Identifying scheduled and unscheduled flows and performing time-based analyses for each group and subgrouping will allow you to determine whether natural and/or artificial variability is the source of the patterns uncovered. Appropriate analyses should be performed to establish whether patient flow problems are manifested as delays, waits, cancellations, rejections, and misplacement. Particular attention should be focused on identifying steps in the care delivery process where the resource is shared between different patient flows, such as obstetrical recovery room resources used both by unscheduled patients who undergo vaginal delivery and patients who are scheduled for induction or C-section. You should be looking particularly for ways of demonstrating a correlation or relationship between a pattern of variability, its source, and its impacts (that is, consequences). These types of analyses should be formulated on the basis of careful deliberation and consideration of how patient demand patterns in one service area may affect flow and services in another.

Inpatient Units

Inpatient units are affected by patient flow problems through arrival and departure patterns of the admissions, transfers, and discharges from the unit. The flow into and out of these units can be driven by arrival patterns that are random (patient driven) and/or by provider scheduling practices that can introduce artificial variability. Basic analyses that examine admissions, discharges, and census by date, DOW, and hour of day will reveal variability in patient demand on the units. Where units are destinations for particular types of patients, these basic analyses can be compared with those that examine the timing of particular procedures, admissions, and so on of those demand streams feeding the particular unit under examination. Although upstream factors such as scheduling of procedures or timing of prior care delivery steps will determine the admission pattern to the unit along with availability of the resource (bed), discharge patterns will be influenced by service time and ability to move to the downstream destination. These factors can affect LOS and patient flow through the unit. Where a particular unit is designated for particular types of patients, identifying whether other patient flow streams are admitted to the unit may be useful in drawing attention to possible quality of care concerns (for example, patient misplacement), bottlenecks existing elsewhere, or a potential impact on other services (for example, increased transport demand in moving patients back to preferred units when a bed becomes available).

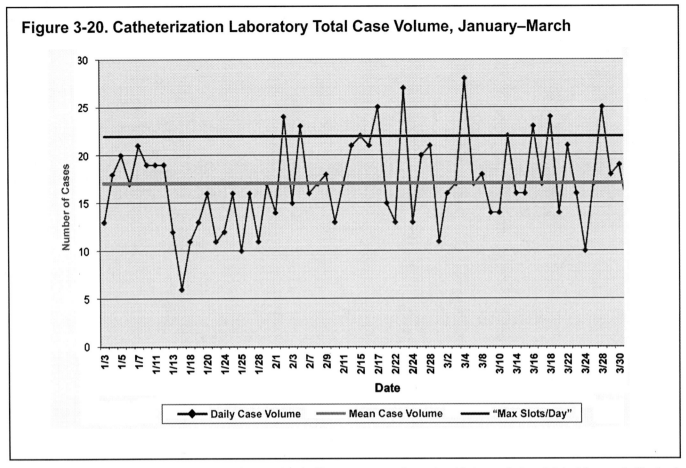

Figure 3-20. Catheterization Laboratory Total Case Volume, January–March

The data, also shown as Figure 3-4, indicate that there can be significant stresses on the system (during peaks in activity) while overall utilization is relatively low. This is a good example of how extreme variability in demand can create alternating periods of stress and low utilization of capacity. The standardized residual (as defined on page 38) is 78%.

When examining patient placement in particular inpatient units, keep in mind that there are likely to be three distinct patient flows relevant to the unit under examination:

1. Patients who should go to the unit and do
2. Patients who should go to the unit but are placed in other units (usually because a bed is not available at the time of admission)
3. Patients who go to the unit but should have gone to another unit (usually because a bed was unavailable there)

Assessing patient flow to and through the ICU is of particular importance because the ICU is a very expensive and critically important service and is typically a shared resource among various patient flow streams. Patient flow problems related to the ICU can have serious quality of care consequences.

Patient-to-Nurse Ratio (PNR)

Patient flow problems affect inpatient units and can have serious quality of care and patient safety consequences (Chapter 2). Inpatient units are generally configured so that they take care of specific types of patients within a defined range of acuity (for example, ICU, surgical step-down, telemetry, medical/surgical). Generally, hospitals staff these units on the basis of a PNR that takes into account the type and acuity of patient being cared for and staff training and experience. Departures from this ratio, which can affect the quality or efficiency of care, can often be traced back to demand variability.

Unit staffing levels can usually be determined from the unit's log or payroll systems. Hospitals normally capture census on their units at least once per day. The number of patients is captured in the unit's census and is affected by both the arrival rate of patients and their LOS on the units. Staffing is usually not static, as hospitals add or lower staffing levels to respond to variable demand.

The patient flow assessment can analyze the PNR, given a unit's census and staffing level at a particular time. Census might be captured only at one or another time during the day. It would be ideal to be able to determine PNR on an hourly basis to capture and measure any short-term fluctuations in PNR, which are less appreciated but no less important.[16] Even when census is captured once a day, calculation of the PNR by date can illustrate whether PNR varies and to what magnitude on the basis of changes in patient demand and/or staffing. For example, Figure 3-21 (below) shows that whereas the average PNR on the unit was about 6:1, the PNR can range from as high as 7.5 to as low as 4:1 on any particular Thursday at noon. Correlation statistics can be applied to the data to determine the strength of the correlation between the PNR and both census and staffing.

The assessment can drill down further by examining the types of patients who make up the census and performing analyses that

examine whether the admission pattern of certain groups of patients, such as elective surgical patients, are driving the variability in PNR (*see* Table 3-2, below).

Ancillary Services

Patients receive a wide range of ancillary services during their stay in the hospital, including radiology and imaging, laboratory, pharmacy, and physical therapy services. The efficiency with which these services are provided and the variability in demand for these services can significantly affect patient flow. Because demand for these services is externally driven, the same variability that drives

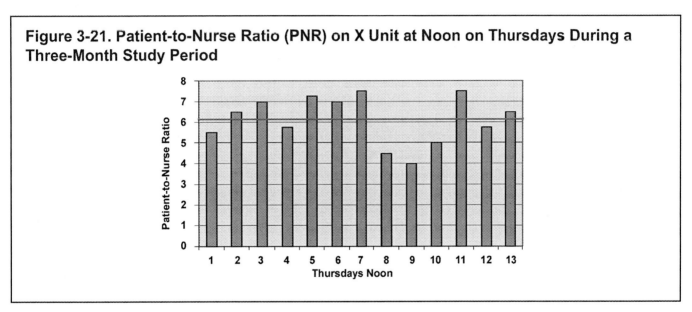

Figure 3-21. Patient-to-Nurse Ratio (PNR) on X Unit at Noon on Thursdays During a Three-Month Study Period

Note the significant and unpredictable variation in PNR across Thursdays (4.0–7.6).

Table 3-2. Patient-to-Nurse Ratio (PNR) Statistics*

| Unit | Correlation Statistic (r) of | | | Max PNR/ Min PNR |
	PNR & No. of Patients	PNR & No. of Nurses	No. of Patients & No. of Nurses	
ICU	.93	.03	.39	2.0
21	.65	−.42	.41	1.7
22	.14	−.71	.57	1.8
23	.69	−.30	.47	1.8
31	.56	−.01	.74	1.7
32	.44	−.53	.53	1.5
33	.44	−.34	.69	1.6

*Max, maximum; min, minimum.

admissions and the timing of operative procedures can affect demand for ancillary services. For example, in an orthopedic clinic setting, the relationship between scheduling of patients, patient arrivals, and radiology testing can be clearly seen in Figure 3-22 (below). Peaks in demand for a particular test or procedure can result in delays in receiving the ancillary service, which in turn can cause delay in downstream services and extended LOS.

The assessment should attempt to determine whether inefficiencies associated with the ancillary service's internal processes result in delays that affect patient flow. Interviews with service staff and major users of the ancillary service can often uncover process issues that result in delays or cancellations.

Patient demand streams, which represent the external force that drives the volume and timing of the testing/procedures, should be the focus of the assessment of ancillary services. Variability should be assessed by examining test and procedure volume by the basic time parameters. After variability is identified, it is important to determine whether it is driven by scheduling practices or whether it is patient driven (for example, as in ED radiology exams). When variability in ancillary service activity reflects variability in patient demand for these services, smoothing of ancillary service activity becomes dependent on addressing variability at the demand source.

Complementary Analyses

As emphasized earlier, the approach for carrying out a hospital-wide patient flow assessment described in this chapter focuses principally on system-level issues. A focus on assessing patient flow beyond the hospital's doors or within a particular hospital service area can represent a complementary (but not an alternative) approach to the one outlined in this chapter.[4] Examining patient flow outside the hospital system itself may well identify opportunities for improving flow in the hospital. For example, a lack of primary care in the community may result in increased readmission rates for certain groups of patients. Assessing and addressing this problem could reduce overall demand for hospital services and thereby alleviate some of the patient flow problems attributed to heightened demand. In addition, assessing coordination with postacute care facilities could identify policies and practices that impede the timely discharge of hospital patients, thereby extending length of stay and contributing to patient flow problems. Such an assessment of patient flow across systems can be beneficial and serve to support the hospitalwide patient flow assessment.

Similarly, assessing patient flow at the service level (for example, in the ED or radiology services) can serve to complement the hospitalwide assessment. Some patient flow practitioners have

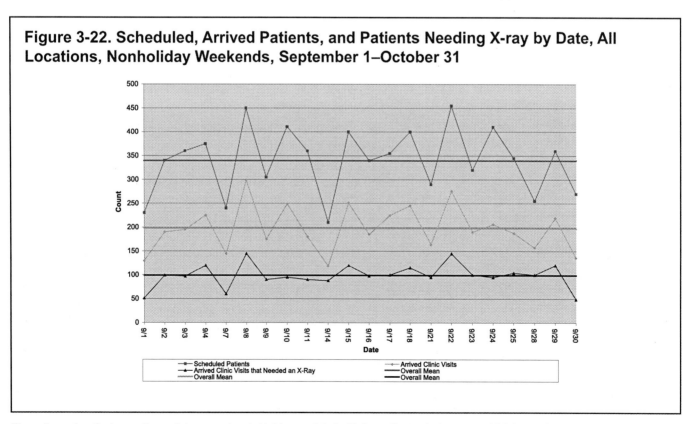

Figure 3-22. Scheduled, Arrived Patients, and Patients Needing X-ray by Date, All Locations, Nonholiday Weekends, September 1–October 31

The pattern of patients needing radiology services is highly correlated with the patient arrival pattern, which in turn is driven by the scheduling of appointments. The difference represents patients who are either no-shows or same-day cancellations.

focused particular attention on assessing the efficiency of patient flow at the interfaces between service areas.[8] Others have narrowed the focus to a comprehensive assessment of flow within a particular service area, such as the perioperative area.[17] Some assessments have used analytic tools and technologies that represent real-time tracking systems or prospective data collection efforts that may be feasible to consider and appropriate for some hospitals considering performing patient flow assessments.

The use of Lean and Six Sigma approaches to analyzing patient flow has been previously mentioned. Process mapping or charting can be valuable not only in identifying the steps in the care delivery process but also in determining non-value-added steps that can be eliminated to thereby improve patient flow.[18,19]

Findings and Developing a Plan of Action

Findings

The analyses in the patient flow assessment yield a set of findings and conclusions regarding the hospital's patient flow problems. These findings and conclusions need to be integrated into a set of recommendations that can provide a blueprint for patient flow improvement. The findings may be numerous and diverse, dealing with patient flow problems that are hospitalwide, apply to cross-service areas, or are limited to process issues within a service area. In addition, the assessment might identify policy, clinical practice, operational, and administrative issues that need to be addressed in the context of patient flow improvement. How do you make sense of the findings that flow from the analyses?

Findings relevant to the goals of the assessment deserve prompt attention. For example, the identification of system-level patient flow bottlenecks is likely to have the greatest impact on hospital patient flow and should be the focus of improvement recommendations. Because of the OR's importance and its impact on both upstream and downstream services, findings pertinent to this area are typically of highest priority. Findings related to the ED may have great importance to the hospital as well because patient flow problems imposed on this service (as well as problems it may impose on itself) can have serious consequences, ranging from poor quality of care to damaged public relations. Other findings may also have a hospitalwide focus and involve changes in policy or practice (for example, creation of an ongoing patient flow committee, changes in physician rounding practices, enforcement of existing admission criteria).

The findings should identify questions and issues that require further exploration. At some point in the assessment process, a decision will have to be made as to whether the goals of the assessment

have been met. Extending the analytic process to examine the myriad additional questions and issues that may arise, especially with regard to operational problems within individual service areas, can be self-defeating if it unduly prolongs the original time lines established for completing the assessment and establishing findings and recommendations and beginning the stage of initiating improvements.

A formal written report should be prepared that presents the analyses, findings, and recommendations. It can have limited or wide circulation; often, an executive summary is prepared for wider distribution. An important consideration is whether individual services should have access to all the analyses, findings, and recommendations or only those pertinent to their service. Because the sources of system-level constraints often lie outside the affected service, however, should sharing of information extend to those services that affect or are affected by the practices of another service? Addressing these issues upfront avoids a later charge that the findings are being "managed" or that the process is less than transparent.

Developing a Plan of Action

The overall goal of the analytic effort is to use the empirical findings of the assessment to formulate recommendations to address patient flow problems and then develop a plan to implement those recommendations. One focus of the recommendations should be how to improve data and IT systems so that patient flow can be assessed on an ongoing basis.

A patient flow assessment should not be viewed as just a one-time undertaking. Bottlenecks are never entirely eliminated in a complex, interconnected system where demand flows are dynamic. Bottlenecks are likely to shift, and assessment of patient flow, like improvement initiatives, should be viewed as a continuous endeavor.

Given the innumerable interconnected and often overlapping care pathways in a typical acute care hospital, a hospitalwide patient flow assessment is likely to identify a range of patient flow problems that need to be addressed. Which problems should be addressed and in what order can be difficult questions to answer. The following considerations may be useful in developing a plan of action on the basis of the following questions:

- Would implementation result in an incremental or full-scale change?
- What would be the impact on system-level problems (as opposed to service-level problems)?
- What are the potential benefits and risks associated with implementing the recommendation?

- What is the potential for successful implementation?
- What is the priority of the problem that would be addressed?
- What is the time line for carrying out the change?
- What resources and "political capital" would be expended to implement the recommendation?
- What is the level of institutional support for the change?

Keeping these questions in mind, a hospital is ready to move forward with devising and adopting strategies for implementing the recommendations and undertaking patient flow improvements, the subject of Chapter 4.

References

1. The Joint Commission: *2009 Comprehensive Accreditation Manual for Hospitals: The Official Handbook.* Oakbrook Terrace, IL: Joint Commission Resources, 2008.

2. The Joint Commission: *Managing Patient Flow: Strategies and Solutions or Addressing Hospital Overcrowding.* Oakbrook Terrace, IL: Joint Commission Resources, 2004.

3. American Hospital Association (AHA): *Hospitals in Pursuit of Excellence.* http://www.ahaqualitycenter.org/qualitycenter/hpoe/content/intro.pdf (accessed Jul. 9, 2009).

4. Vissers J., Beech R (eds.): *Health Operations Management: Patient Flow Logistics in Health Care.* New York: Routledge, 2005.

5. Litvak E., Long M.C.: Cost and quality under managed care: Irreconcilable differences? *Am J Manag Care* 3:305–312, Mar. 2000.

6. Kane R.L., et al.: *Nurse Staffing and Quality of Patient Care.* Evidence Report/Technology Assessment No. 151, Mar. 2007. http://www.ahrq.gov/downloads/pub/evidence/pdf/nursestaff/nursestaff.pdf (accessed Jul. 14, 2009).

7. Young T., et al.: Using industrial processes to improve patient care. *BMJ* 328:162–164, Jan. 17, 2004.

8. Hall R.W., et al.: Modeling patient flows through the health care system. In Hall R.W. (ed.): *Flow: Reducing Delay in Healthcare Delivery.* New York: Springer, 2006.

9. Trusko B.E., et al.: *Improving Healthcare Quality and Cost with Six Sigma.* Upper Saddle River, NJ: FT Press, 2007.

10. DeFrances C.J., Cullen K.A., Kozak L.J.: National Hospital Discharge Survey: 2005 annual summary with detailed diagnosis and procedure data. *Vital Health Stat 13* 165:1–209, Dec. 2007.

11. Allen S.: Getting with the flow helps hospital deliver service. *Boston Globe,* Jan. 25, 2005. http://www.boston.com/news/local/articles/2005/01/25/getting_with_the_flow_helps_hospital_deliver_service/ (accessed Jul. 14, 2009).

12. Kolker A.: Process modeling of ICU patient flow: Effect of daily load leveling of elective surgeries on ICU diversion. *J Med Syst* 33:27–40, Feb. 2009.

13. Welch S.J.: The emergency department performance measures and benchmarking summit. *Emergency Medicine News* 28:24–25, Jun. 2006. http://journals.lww.com/em-news/Fulltext/2006/06000/The_Emergency_Department_Performance_Measures_and.19.aspx (accessed Oct. 19, 2009).

14. Medical Connectivity: *National Patient Flow Survey—2008,* Feb. 5, 2009. http://medicalconnectivity.com/2009/02/05/national-patient-flow-survey-2008/ (accessed Jul. 14, 2009).

15. Program for Management of Variability in Health Care Delivery: *Improving Patient Flow and Throughput in California Hospitals Operating Room Services.* Prepared for the California Healthcare Foundation, 2007, Chapters 5 and 6. http://www.bu.edu/mvp/Library/CHCF%20Guidance%20document.pdf (accessed Jul. 14, 2009).

16. Fuda K.K., et al.: Short-term variability in patient-to-nurse ratios: Extent and causes (unpublished manuscript). Boston, Mar. 2009.

17. Rotondi A.J., et al.: Benchmarking the perioperative process. I. Patient routing systems: A method for continual improvement of patient flow and resource utilization. *J Clin Anesth* 9:159–169, Mar. 1997.

18. Smith B.: Lean and Six Sigma: A one-two punch. *Quality Progress* 36:37–41, Apr. 2003.

19. Institute for Healthcare Improvement: *Going Lean in Health Care.* IHI Innovation Series white paper. Cambridge, MA: Institute for Healthcare Improvement, 2005 (available on www.IHI.org; accessed Sep. 11, 2009).

Chapter 4

Strategies for Managing Patient Flow

Sandeep Green Vaswani, M.B.A.; Michael C. Long, M.D.; Brad Prenney, M.S., M.P.A.; Eugene Litvak, Ph.D.

R ecently, for reasons discussed elsewhere (*see* Chapters 1 and 2), improvement of patient flow has become a universal goal in health care. As a consequence, consultants and others have promoted a variety of approaches to patient flow management. In this chapter, we review some of the most common patient flow management strategies and, more importantly, focus on what we believe is the core foundation for patient flow management. Most industries methodically study and manage the flow of materials, data, or customers on the basis of the multidisciplinary science of operations management (OM), also called operations research. We start with an overview of key principles of patient flow management strategy and then provide a brief background on OM. We then introduce variability methodology (VM), which plays a critical role in allowing us to appropriately employ traditional OM methodologies such as queuing and simulation. We devote the main body of the chapter to a detailed description of a multiphase approach to patient flow redesign based on OM/VM. Finally, we review other tools that can help with patient flow management and suggest how to use them to complement the improvements from OM/VM.

The focus of this chapter is on the flow of patients throughout a hospital—broader than just the typical scrutiny of flow on inpatient units but limited to the confines of a typical hospital. That said, as stated in the Introduction (page xii), the concepts presented are just as applicable to postacute settings such as rehabilitation and skilled nursing facilities, as well as other health care delivery organizations, such as freestanding emergency departments (EDs), laboratories, primary care practices, and ambulatory care centers.

Key Principles of Any Strategy to Manage Patient Flow

Systemwide Rather Than Silos

The first and most important principle of a patient flow management strategy is that it take a systemwide view instead of a departmental (including unit-level) or other narrow view. Health care delivery organizations tend to be departmentally oriented. One reason is the high level of subspecialization in every segment of care, which makes for different operational characteristics in every department. Other than the flow of patients from and to other departments, all departments function as independent microcosms. Departmental performance is reviewed, and managers are rewarded by how well each hospital unit minimizes cost per unit of service and maximizes utilization of its own specific resources. These incentives can result in behaviors that are counterproductive to maximizing systemwide patient flow.

For example, a housekeeping manager's goal may be to minimize the amount of time that his or her staff is not busy. One result of pursuing such a goal would be high utilization of housekeeping staff and, arguably, low cost per unit of services provided by the housekeeping department. Another result would be a higher frequency of times when housekeeping personnel are not available. This would lead to delays in other departments seeking housekeeping services. For example, the delay in turning around an inpatient-unit bed can then delay a patient's move out of the ED or the OR recovery area. Delays in moving patients out of the ED or OR can cause those beds and resources to become fully occupied, which in turn can delay moving patients into the ED (from registration/waiting) or the OR. The "super" efficiency of one department can inadvertently impose a significant cascading inefficiency and increased cost on the overall health care system. *The most important goal of patient flow strategy should be to maximize patient throughput (number of patients per time unit) while simultaneously minimizing overall resources needed to serve those patients within clinically acceptable wait times and with high quality of care.* With this system goal in mind, individual departments' goals should be designed first to serve the systemwide patient flow goal and then to maximize every department's own efficiency. In case of conflict (for example, maximize flow through the operating room [OR] versus flow through an ICU), a hospital will need to make trade-offs on the basis of its unique circumstances and goals.

Science-Based and Data-Driven

The next most important principle of a patient flow management strategy is that it be based in OM science and rigorous data analysis. Management decisions are often made on the basis of instinct (a classic example is the building of a larger emergency room to address ED overcrowding when the real problem is elsewhere, as explained at greater length on page 63) or as a compromise between demands from competing departments (often the loudest wins) and resource constraints. If data analysis is conducted, it often focuses on maximizing departmental goals, such as maximization of the housekeeper utilization rate, as cited in the earlier example, at the expense of system impact. Another issue that an assessment helps to shed light on, as described in Chapter 3, is that every hospital's patient flow problems can be unique, depending on that hospital's operational structures. Patient flow strategy has to take these idiosyncrasies into account. For example, consider two different ICUs, one with 5 beds and another with

10. Let's say that the first ICU faces a demand of 1 admission per day and that the second has a demand of 2 admissions per day. Both ICUs have the same average length of stay (LOS) of 2.5 days. What would be the likelihood that a bed will not be available when a patient arrives at each of the two ICUs? Because the demand is twice as much for the unit with twice as many beds, it may seem that the probability of no bed being available would be similar. On the contrary, the probability that no bed will be available for the 5-bed ICU is higher—not just a little higher but as much as three times higher than for the 10-bed ICU.[1] This is why simplistic comparison of seemingly similar units can be quite misleading. OM science offers a multitude of tools, such as queuing models (which is how the above probabilities were estimated), simulation, and optimization to address patient flow issues. When deployed properly, these tools enable accurate planning of resources to attain required service levels (for example, wait times, bed availability for certain types of patients). OM science also allows for considered decision making in the context of conflicts (such as the trade-off between housekeeper utilization and bed turnover time) and constraints. This is very important in health care, where operations tend to be quite complicated compared with those in other industries. Finally, scientifically based and data-driven design is objective, with specific, measurable performance metrics, and hence more likely to receive buy-in from physicians.

The Right Structure Before Improving Microprocesses

Health care delivery presents opportunities for improvement in many facets of its operations. Improvements are possible in the flow of patients through various parts of a hospital's care delivery system, as well as in microprocesses such as the delivery of individual services such as laboratory tests, diagnostic imaging, procedures performed on patients in an inpatient unit, and so on. Although improving existing microprocesses can yield benefits, some of the key patient flow–related issues are fundamentally structural in nature. For example, improving the preadmission process for surgical patients can no doubt improve flow by reducing cancellations and patient-driven delays. However, it would not address structural issues such as how different types of surgeries are scheduled and how OR resources are organized for different types of surgical flows. Another example of microprocess improvement is the frequent expenditure of time and effort on continually improving (that is, decreasing) turnover time between surgical cases. However, if insufficient time is freed up to add another case to the operating day, there is no improvement in OR throughput—and the premise of the focus on turnover time is called into question. In comparison, addressing structural issues, such as by separating inpatient and outpatient surgeries (where appropriate), can have a much more substantive impact on turnover times and overall OR throughput. Addressing structure is significantly more critical to patient flow strategy than merely improving individual processes because the major source of patient flow problems is variability in patient demand, as described in greater detail later in this chapter. In addition, fixing structural issues could alter microprocesses and the improvement needs therein. In other words, ignoring structure and addressing microprocesses could turn out to be wasted effort when structure is subsequently addressed (for example, OR turnover would need to be reevaluated after inpatient and outpatient surgery areas were separated).

A Compliance Review and Enforcement Process

Because old practices die hard and because of the day-to-day fluidity of flow in health care, it is imperative that any patient flow strategy have compliance review as an essential component. Compliance review helps manage and resolve the conflicting priorities and tensions between system goals and those of individual departments or services. Without periodic review and enforcement of policies, one can always find a reason to violate one or more rules, depending on the circumstances. For example, a telemetry unit might have specific admission criteria, but if one physician has a preference for that unit for nonclinical reasons (such as a desire to locate his patients together or because the unit is newer than others), he might manipulate the admission process to get his patient admitted there. If repeat violations go unchecked, their volume would tend to increase over time. One offense may result in others feeling the inequity and engaging in similar activity. Quickly, the entire system is threatened. The role of compliance review is to maintain the integrity and fairness of a system and to identify gaps in the system that need to be addressed. Some compliance review activity can occur after the fact (within a reasonable period of time), while other compliance discussions may need to occur in the moment. For example, whether a particular patient is appropriate for admission to a specific unit may be in the gray zone for that unit's admission criteria, and someone needs to have the authority to arbitrate that situation in real time (*see* "Conducting Compliance Review," page 67).

A Brief Background on Operations Management

Addressing patient flow without employing OM methods is unlikely to yield lasting results. OM, "the use of quantitative methods to assist analysts and decision-makers in designing, analyzing, and improving the performance or operation of systems,"[2(p. 1)] began as a formal discipline during World War II, driven by military needs to allocate scarce resources toward attaining specific goals. It has since been applied extensively in industry, including manufacturing, transportation, and finance. Over time, the scientific techniques of OM have continued to evolve, driven by application to increasingly complex operational problems and the advent of high-speed computers, which make it feasible to perform complicated mathematical calculations within very short periods. The application of OM is described as follows:

> Mathematical, computational, and analytical tools and devices are employed merely to provide information and insight into systems and processes; and ultimately, it is the human decision makers who will utilize and implement what has been learned through the analysis process to achieve the most favorable performance of the system.[2(p. 1)]

OM science is now a field unto itself, with its own graduate-level courses and doctoral programs. Given the scope of this chapter, we now highlight the OM methodologies that are most pertinent to patient flow management:

- **Critical path method:** A technique primarily used for planning projects with many interdependent activities, the critical path method can be applied to any health care process to identify key points of handoff (handover) and to organize resources to minimize delays and the length of time a patient spends in the overall process.
- **Queuing theory:** Queuing theory has been described as follows:

> …the study of waiting in various guises. It uses queuing models to represent the various types of queuing systems (systems that involve waiting in lines of some kind) that arise in practice. Formulas for each model indicate how the corresponding queuing system should perform, including the average amount of waiting that will occur, under a variety of circumstances.[3(p. 765)]

The ED and other areas with urgent arrivals to a hospital are excellent candidates for application of queuing theory. For example, it can be used to determine the resources needed to ensure a 30-minute door-to-doctor time in the ED.

- **Simulation:** Simulation is used in industry to prospectively explore the effects of alternate designs, particularly for complex systems with many variables and interrelationships. First, a model is built to mimic a particular flow or process. A very important, and often overlooked, next step is to validate the model by ensuring that it accurately replicates current experience. Once that is done, the model can be used to test new permutations and combinations of inputs to maximize desired outcomes while minimizing costs and to test the effects of various system constraints. Although simulation is perhaps most relevant to health care, with its complex interconnected operations, health care is also the industry least developed in terms of application.[4]

Why Hasn't Health Care Widely Adopted Operations Management?

There are many reasons why health care has not adopted OM as widely as have other industries. First, a hospital is not a manufacturing organization. The mixing of material and people flow, subjective output products, and complex line of command, for example, all make hospitals different from manufacturing organizations.[5] Historically, cost-plus reimbursement for health care services has not created motivation to improve the efficiency and quality of care delivery. Second, despite the vast amount of data collected in hospitals, there remains a paucity of reliable operational data, such as clinical urgency with a specific time limit (for example, 4 hours, 24 hours) and time stamps capturing a patient's progression (for example, a patient was ready to be admitted from the ED at 4:10 P.M. (16:10) and actually left at 6:42 P.M. (18:42). Third, traditional OM techniques cannot be applied to health care in a cookie-cutter fashion. For example, overbooking is a well-accepted tool for managing demand in the face of last-minute cancellations. Airlines frequently use overbooking to maximize occupancy on flights. When airlines have to turn away a few ticketed passengers from a flight, they compensate them with hotel stays, free airline tickets, and so on. But imagine applying overbooking in a surgical setting. On some days, the hospital would have to cancel a patient's elective surgery because of lack of availability of resources (for example, room, surgeon, staff). What could be offered to that patient as compensation? Another procedure for free? A free day in the ICU? You can see how simplistically borrowing techniques from other industries may not work for health care.

More fundamentally, in health care, different types of patient flows—some controllable, others not—put demands on a system with relatively fixed capacity. The problem is that these two types of flows have different service requirements. The controllable flow to a hospital (elective and scheduled) needs to be serviced in the most efficient manner to maximize the utilization of hospital resources and overall throughput of such cases. The most important need of uncontrollable (emergency and urgent) flows to a hospital is to provide care within a clinically appropriate waiting time. To further complicate matters, the uncontrollable flows (for example, ED patients) cannot altogether be turned away from the system without compromising quality of care. In contrast, a restaurant may take reservations as well as walk-ins. When the wait time for a table becomes excessive, some walk-in patrons will just go away. Compare that with a hospital, where some patients are scheduled arrivals while others arrive unannounced. While hospitals can and do go on diversion, arguably excessively, the effect of delays in receiving care is far greater than that of a delayed meal.

Any business that can control—that is, schedule—its inflows typically does so to maximize its throughput. Hospitals, on the other hand, have not had much success in managing controllable inflows[6] because efforts to do so often conflict with provider practices and priorities. For example, surgeons and cardiologists typically are given block time in ORs or cardiac catheterization laboratories, which they are free to schedule into, generally without regard for consequences for inpatient units or other clinical services. Mixing of controllable (but unmanaged) and uncontrollable inflows in hospital operations makes it impossible to apply traditional OM methods to overall patient flow. Applying certain queuing models to mixed flows that are not random is inappropriate because the models frequently assume statistically random arrivals, which is not the case with mixed flows. Moreover, the part of the flow that is controllable can be serviced with fewer resources than would be predicted by a queuing model, and so using queuing for overall flows can lead to inefficiency and waste of health care resources. In summary, health care by nature and practice has not lent itself to the application of traditional OM methodologies.

Variability Methodology

To address the particular nuances of hospital patient flow, faculty of the newly created nonprofit Institute for Healthcare Optimization (IHO; previously Boston University's Program for Management of Variability in Healthcare Delivery [MVP]) developed variability methodology (VM).[6,7] VM is not a proprietary methodology. It is described quite extensively in a report prepared for the California Healthcare Foundation in 2007.[7] One of IHO's main goals is to widely disseminate OM and VM for health care improvement. At its core, VM entails identifying variability in every step of the care delivery process, as described in Chapter 3, and then separating the different types of variability to design operations systems to address each appropriately. An ideal health care system is one where capacity is just sufficient to meet demand for service at every step in the care delivery process. When patient demand is variable, the health care system is challenged to align or adjust its capacity in a timely manner to service that demand. Eliminating variability where you can and optimally managing it when you can't eliminate it is the fundamental starting point of optimally managing patient flow. An entire book can be, and perhaps should be, written about VM and its applications in health care alone.

We now provide a summary overview of key VM principles and how they can be used to devise strategies for hospital patient flow management. Although this summary does not comprehensively cover all aspects of VM and its implications, the following material should be adequate for any hospital trying to redesign its operations to maximize patient flow. Implementing the recommendations outlined in the following sections is predicated on a hospital's resources for operations data analysis, clinical expertise, and organizational change management. These three resources are like legs of a stool that provide the necessary foundation for patient flow design and management. If a hospital lacks resources in one of these three areas, it may well choose to engage outside consultants, but we would suggest one caveat—that the consultants have the necessary training and skills to fully understand and facilitate the changes as described.

Different Types of Variability in Health Care Delivery

If all patients arrived uniformly over time, had the same disease, and experienced exactly the same recovery, and if all clinicians had the same ability to provide care, it would be possible to design a 100% efficient patient flow process. This is obviously not reality. Even patients with the same disease experience different levels of illness and have different responses to treatment. This type of variation is called *clinical variability*. Patients do not arrive for care at a uniform rate but rather whenever the need arises. This is *flow variability*. Finally, care providers are not uniform in their ability to provide quality care. For example, different surgeons take different amounts of time to perform the same procedure, even if all else is the same. This type of variation is called *professional variability*. These three types of variability are naturally occurring, and unless interfered with, they typically follow random statistical patterns.

The presence of natural variability—as clinical, flow, and professional variability—makes it impossible to design patient flow operations that are 100% efficient and that simultaneously deliver the highest possible quality. Such systems by definition will not become a Toyota product line and will need to be less than 100% efficient so that they reliably provide a required level of service (for example, limited waiting time) and high-quality care. Queuing and other traditional OM methods can be used to design systems to manage natural variability. However, the problem is that health care is beset not just with different forms of natural variability but also a number of artificially introduced variabilities.

What Is Artificial Variability, and Where Does It Come From?

Artificial variability arises out of inadvertence, provider scheduling practices, and/or inappropriate management of patient flow. It is present to some extent in every patient's journey through the hospital. For example, two patients with similar diseases and recovery may spend very different amounts of time in an ICU because of downstream-bed availability; one patient may be able to move to a medical/surgical unit as soon as he or she is clinically ready, whereas another might have to stay in the ICU for a few hours or even days longer than clinically necessary. This extended LOS represents artificial variability but could easily be confused with naturally occurring clinical variability. Take the example of two patients requiring a standard surgical procedure. Let's say that both patients have very similar manifestations but are operated on by two different surgeons. Even if both surgeons take exactly the same amount of time, one patient may end up in the OR longer than the other if the OR went on hold in one case because of unavailability of a postanesthesia care unit (PACU) bed. Such a variation in case length could be inappropriately classified as natural professional variability, whereas the real cause is artificial in nature.

The most significant artificial variability from a patient flow perspective is introduced by dysfunctional scheduling of elective admissions in to a hospital. Unlike emergency and urgent patients, such elective patients provide a longer window of time for treatment to begin. This demand for hospital services can be arranged so as to maximize efficiency and throughput. Unfortunately, current scheduling practices for elective admissions do not attempt to benefit from the longer acceptable wait times for these patients. On the contrary, current scheduling practices allow elective case variability frequently to exceed what would appear with arrivals through the ED (*see* Figure 4-1, page 62). This effect was first identified by Litvak and Long[6] and later documented in other publications.[8]

If you ask any ED administrator how many admissions to plan for, say, on a Wednesday in three weeks, you will likely get a quick and pretty accurate response (barring major calamities). Ask the same question of a surgery administrator, and he or she will likely have no idea. Why is that the case when surgery typically has a large proportion of schedulable elective cases? Artificial variability, as compared with natural variability, is nonrandom, "yet it also is unpredictable, driven by numerous competing demands on the surgeons' time that are usually unknown and therefore unaccounted for by the healthcare system."[6(p. 308)]

The Effects of Artificial Variability

Any variability increases cost and reduces efficiency. Although some of the negative effects now described may also result from natural variability, most of the variability that causes severe system dysfunction is artificial in nature. Natural variability needs to be managed to optimize levels of quality and service (for more details, *see* "The Only Solution for Artificial Variability: Variability Methodology," page 63). *Artificial variability cannot be predicted or managed but must be investigated and eliminated.*

Figure 4-1. Admissions from Emergency Department (ED) Versus Elective AM Admissions from the Operating Room (OR)

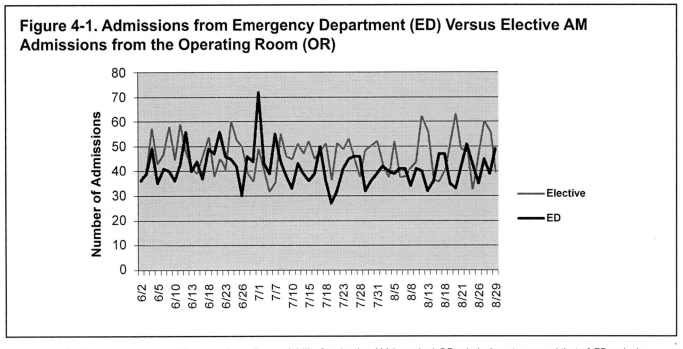

As shown in the figure, current scheduling practices allow variability for elective AM (morning) OR admissions to exceed that of ED arrivals.
Source: *Palmetto Health Richland, Columbia, South Carolina. Used with permission.*

Compromised Quality of Care. Artificial variability reduces quality in several ways. For example, peaks in elective flows lead to enhanced peaks in inpatient unit census. Variability in census in turn leads to variability in nurse-to-patient staffing ratios. It has been established that decreases in these ratios results in increased mortality; and mortality increases more steeply as the ratio continues to decline[9,10] (*see* Chapter 2). This decrease in quality is directly imposed on the system by artificial variability in elective admission patterns. Other effects of artificial variability that reduce quality of care include patient misplacement because of a lack of appropriate inpatient beds at the right time; increased ED waiting and boarding due to competition with elective admissions, especially on peak elective days; increased waits for urgent surgeries; and increased PACU boarding.[11,12]

Decreased Patient Satisfaction. Artificial variability causes patients to wait longer than they otherwise would. For example, on peak elective admission days, ED patients are forced to wait for a prolonged period because of the reduced availability of inpatient beds. On the other hand, an emergent surgical case coming from the ED could upend the day's elective schedule in the OR, leading to bumping, with delayed elective cases being done late in the evening. Although patient expectations have been set to accept emergency-driven delays, prolonged waits, uncertainty, and being NPO (nothing by mouth) for excessive time do not drive high marks from patients. Similarly, long waits in the ED unrelated to the care process do not garner high satisfaction scores.[13]

Decreased Provider and Staff Satisfaction. Clinical work is hard enough if providers and staff have only to deal with the natural variability in health care. Artificial variability has the effect of increasing the pressure in an already stressed system by adding more and greater peaks and valleys in demand, along with a measure of unpredictability. The end result is increased use of overtime and nursing float pool staff. In addition, providers and staff are regularly faced with significant peaks and valleys in workload, which not only affects the quality of care and patient satisfaction, as described, but also staff and provider quality of work–life balance, job satisfaction, and staff retention.

Operational Inefficiency/High Cost of Care. Another important effect of artificial variability is the increase in the cost of care. Artificial variability reduces the number of patients a hospital can care for with existing resources. Let's look at an example to illustrate this point. Say that you know you have to provide care for five patients a day, and it takes one hour per patient to provide requisite services. In one scenario, you can schedule these patients any way you like. In another scenario, someone else controls when these patients arrive; that person does not tell you when he or she will send the patients, but you are required to provide services as soon as they arrive. In the first case, you can choose to staff for five hours of your choosing and provide care to all of these patients. In the second scenario, you would have to be prepared throughout the day to provide care for the same patients. Clearly, the first scenario would be more efficient. However, the latter is not far from what happens in ORs and cardiac catheterization laboratories where elective cases are treated. With inpatient occupancy averaging 65% in the United States in 2007,[14] even if one assumes that the entire patient demand is naturally distributed (that is, no elective admissions), then according to queuing theory, increasing occupancy to 80% is quite possible without compromising access. When there is a significant elective component in admissions (the most typical case), occupancy can well exceed 90%. In fact, short of further increasing health care costs, smoothing artificial variability is the only way to increase bed occupancy without compromising access to care.[1] The financial benefit of increasing occupancy in the hospitals in the United States could be substantial enough to address the health care needs of the millions of uninsured and underinsured. Although outside the scope of this chapter, smoothing of artificial variability has significant health policy implications as well, such as the needs for the capacity to increase access for the under- and uninsured and for an aging population and for the clinical staff to support growing demand (is there a real shortage, or is it inefficiency?), as well as the question of how to achieve safe nursing staffing levels.

Role of Variability Methodology in Patient Flow Strategy

During the past few years, the health care system in the United States appears to have increasingly approached its capacity ceiling. Hospitals, particularly EDs, report being overwhelmed by patient demand.[15] A recent U.S. General Accountability Office (GAO) report calls attention to inpatient bed unavailability as a key driver of ED overcrowding. As stated in the report, "we found that one key factor contributing to crowding was the availability of inpatient beds for patients admitted to the hospital from the emergency department."[16] These capacity issues have turned the spotlight on patient flow management as a method for increasing hospital efficiency and throughput. Hospital construction was also increasing until the credit market dried up in 2008,[17] making patient flow management even more important. *Optimal management of artificial variability in demand can virtually increase the effective capacity of an individual hospital and the overall health care system without the commensurate addition of resources.* The Institute of Medicine has recognized the importance of variability methodology and OM science in the following recommendation:

> By applying variability methodology, queuing theory and the inputs—transformation—outputs model, hospitals can identify and eliminate many of the patient flow impediments caused by operational inefficiencies.[15(p. 135–136)]

Let us examine how VM works, using the example of ED overcrowding. Several studies have recognized the lack of inpatient beds as the main cause of ED overcrowding.[16,18,19] As a result, several hospitals have decided to add inpatient beds. At first blush, this appears to be a reasonable action. Yet hospitals then face the question of how many to add. When artificial variability is present, there is no analytic approach to answer this question. Moreover, inpatient bed unavailability is often a periodic phenomenon rather than a permanent one; that is, beds are available for ED patients on certain days of the week or times of the day and not others. What this means is that an overall shortage of beds is not the true root cause of ED overcrowding. So what drives ED overcrowding? What causes beds to be more available for ED patients on certain days than on others? What kinds of patients are occupying more beds on certain days than on others? One study, using data from two Massachusetts hospitals, has demonstrated that peaks in scheduled admissions are the main determinant of ED overcrowding.[18] The recent GAO report states the following: "One reason for a lack of access to inpatient beds is competition between hospital admissions from the emergency department and scheduled admissions—for example, for elective surgeries, which may be more profitable for the hospital."[16] The main reason that there are peaks in scheduled admissions is artificial variability created by dysfunctional scheduling of elective admissions. Any attempt to improve patient flow without addressing this artificial variability results in a temporary improvement at best. Artificial variability wreaks havoc not only on the flow of scheduled admissions but on many other parts of the health care delivery process, as discussed earlier, resulting in higher health care costs overall.

The Only Solution for Artificial Variability: Variability Methodology

There are no known scientific approaches to designing an operations infrastructure to efficiently deal with artificial variability. Any ad hoc attempt to do so will eventually fail because of the intrinsic unpredictability of artificial variability. *The only approach to "managing" artificial variability is to eliminate it altogether.* The first step in this process is to *identify* variability in the area under study. Typically this is done using a chart displaying changes in a metric (for example, volume) over time. The variation over time is then *classified* as either natural or artificial variability. A simple statistical test of randomness can be helpful to ascertain whether variation in the metric is random and thus naturally occurring (*see* Sidebar 5-1, Chapter 5). That said, health care is fraught with examples in which seemingly random variability is actually artificial, as already indicated.[20] So, regardless of the results of the statistical randomness test, it is important to consider all possible sources of variation. If there is no apparent natural reason for the variability to be present, then it is likely to have been artificially introduced by human decisions.[20] Variability that is nonrandom and at the same time not predictable is clearly artificial. After variability has been identified and classified, it needs to be *quantified*—as the deviation from an ideal expected pattern. For many systems under scrutiny, the sum of the absolute differences of individual data points from the mean (sum of residuals) is an appropriate measure of variability. The final step is to *eliminate*, or *significantly decrease*, all artificial variability through system redesign and then manage any remaining natural variability.

A key concept in managing natural variability is the separation of homogenous subgroups on the basis of clinical and/or operational characteristics so as to maximize efficiency and throughput. An example of separate homogenous subgroups is fast-track versus high-acuity ED patients. Although all these patients enter the ED through the same portal, some patients present with lower-acuity issues that require less testing and more routine treatment. They have a clearly distinct clinical profile from that of the higher-acuity patients. Assigning these patients to a fast-track system can significantly increase provider efficiency and patient flow efficiency for these patients as well as for the ED overall. In general, separation of patient flows into homogenous groups allows for higher efficiency for that group, which in turn enables higher overall efficiency of the system.

How far do you subdivide into homogenous subgroups? From an operational efficiency perspective, the formation of a subgroup must be based on two key criteria: expectations of improved quality and lower cost. "Super" subspecialization is virtually a force of nature in health care these days. With the development of interdisciplinary specialties, hospitals sometimes provide exactly the same services under multiple divisions. The reasons for doing so are often related to provider preference and not clinically driven. For example, you can have an echocardiogram from cardiology or from radiology just 100 yards apart, with each department having its own equipment and staff for this test. Apart from being confusing for referring physicians and patients, such a practice does nothing for operational efficiency unless each has sufficient patient flow to justify the existence of the testing capability. The ideal in patient care may be a subgroup of one, where every patient is treated uniquely, with all services designed to revolve around each patient. However, the cost of this ideal system would be astronomical. Instead, homogenous groups should be subdivided until the two criteria of quality and cost are optimized and the remaining flows are treated as one group for the purposes of operations and flow redesign.

A Three-Phase Approach to Redesign of Patient Flow Management

As discussed, an important driver of hospitalwide patient flow issues is the flow of electively admitted patients. Typically, surgical patients constitute fewer than half of admitted patients for many hospitals. Although the proportion of surgical patients that is elective varies across hospitals, elective surgeries are frequently the biggest source of artificial variability in patient flow across the hospital. Hospitals with cardiac catheterization laboratories also experience significant artificial flow variability from their elective cases. Some hospitals may also have a significant level of scheduled medical admissions, particularly for cancer services. Obstetrics is another service composed of scheduled and unscheduled flows, and the principles and phased approach that we now describe also have direct application in managing patient flow for this service. For all these reasons, *any patient flow improvement strategy has to have at its foundation the separation of elective and unscheduled flows and the elimination of artificial variability in elective patient flow.* To achieve this, the three-phase approach (*see* Figure 4-2, page 65) was developed by Boston University's MVP.

In Phase 1, which involves classification and separation of flows, dedicated resources are set aside for urgent/emergent and semielective flows, especially in the OR and cardiac catheterization laboratory but also in other units with a significant mix of elective and nonelective patients. The reason for separation of resources is that the management objectives are different for each of these flows. The most important goal for the urgent and semielective flows is timely access to services; the most important goal for the elective flow is the maximization of efficiency and volume. These goals can be achieved only by providing dedicated separate resources for each flow, assuming that the volume of each is sufficient to warrant allocation of separate resources. In addition, phase 1 involves separation of day-surgery cases from inpatient cases if each flow is high enough to warrant its own resources. The reason, again, is to maximize efficiency and throughput for those two categories of cases; even though both are electively scheduled, they have significant clinical and management differences. After elective inpatient flows have been clearly identified and separated in Phase 1, it becomes possible, in Phase 2, to redesign these flows by smoothing the daily demand pattern from the OR or catheterization laboratory for appropriate destination units, while taking into account variation in LOS, to reduce day-to-day variability in the number of admissions and/or unit census. Smoothing maximizes the utilization of inpatient resources and minimizes the competition between elective flows and ED admissions for inpatient beds. Finally, after separating and smoothing elective flows, bed and staffing needs can be accurately determined in Phase 3 of redesign.

Each of the three phases is discussed in more detail in turn. Although the three-phase approach can be applied to any major source of admissions to a hospital, such as the OR and the cardiac catheterization laboratory, it is not limited to those areas. Artificial

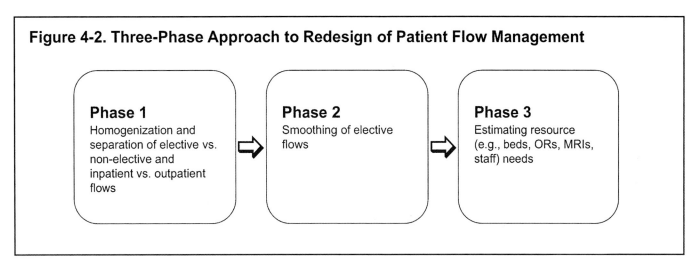

Figure 4-2. Three-Phase Approach to Redesign of Patient Flow Management

Phase 1
Homogenization and separation of elective vs. non-elective and inpatient vs. outpatient flows

Phase 2
Smoothing of elective flows

Phase 3
Estimating resource (e.g., beds, ORs, MRIs, staff) needs

The three-phase approach to redesign of patient flow management entails the separation of elective and unscheduled flows and the elimination of artificial variability in elective patient flow. OR, operating room; MRI, magnetic resonance imaging.

variability can be found throughout the health care delivery spectrum—such as in clinics, laboratories, and procedural areas—and should be rooted out with a thorough rigorous application of the three-phase approach no matter where it is found. Nonetheless, for the purposes of this chapter, we focus on the OR because the magnitude of its impact on overall hospital flow makes it a necessary foundation for patient flow management.

Phase 1: Homogenization and Separation of Elective and Nonelective Flows

Establishing an Objective Urgency Classification System. The first step in Phase 1 is to classify cases by urgency at the time of scheduling. The following three major patient flows should be identified:

- Urgent/emergent (unscheduled)
- Work-in
- Elective

Hospital data systems often have an existing data field that is used to mark cases as "elective," "urgent,'" or "emergent," but this field may be arbitrarily populated by various personnel and is frequently inaccurate. In addition, the existing urgency classification may not have any specific time limit associated with it. How soon does an urgent/emergent case need to get done? Can all urgent cases wait the same amount of time before outcomes deteriorate? Finally, existing data may not represent the urgency at the time the case presented; they may have been modified after the fact for a variety of reasons (sometimes urgency is populated by medical records staff on the basis of admission source or the type of procedure that was performed, neither of which accurately reflects the precise urgency at the time of booking). What is required is a prospective (at the time of scheduling), surgeon-driven classification system

that has very specific time limits associated with each urgency category. There are no hard-and-fast rules as to what the urgency classification should look like, but the following principles should be incorporated into the urgency classification system:

1. It is very important that surgeons develop their own classification on the basis of case mix and clinically appropriate practice patterns. Some life-and-death emergencies will typically be classified as needing access to the OR within 30 minutes. Other cases are able to wait longer, and acceptable waiting times may vary from hospital to hospital. There is no right answer, but it is important that each surgeon community at each hospital reach consensus for each type of case as to the maximal clinically acceptable waiting time for each urgency grouping.

2. The total number of urgency groupings should not be more than five to seven to simplify use of the system (*see* Table 4-1, page 66, and Chapter 6 for examples of urgency groupings). In addition to unscheduled procedures that must get OR access within 24 hours, hospitals usually have a number of work-in or add-on procedures that are semielective (*see* "Separating Work-in Flow," page 67) and need to be scheduled within a few days. This group of work-in cases is often overlooked in the OR schedule design, which can potentially result in delays and quality/safety concerns. All other procedures are purely elective in that there is significant latitude in scheduling timing.

3. Perhaps most importantly, urgency should be based solely on patients' clinical needs. Unscheduled cases (wait time up to 24 hours) are randomly occurring. Basing urgency subdivisions of the unscheduled group solely on clinical needs is the only way to develop a reliable system that is not corrupted by artificial variability. For example, an open fracture may have a maximum clinically driven wait time of eight

hours, but a surgeon may delay these cases to be performed at the end of the day to accommodate an elective schedule in the OR or his or her need to be present in the clinic. Doing so adds significant artificial variability in wait times for these cases. It then becomes impossible to design a reliable system to provide consistent and efficient high-quality care.

After the urgency classification system has been developed, it should be implemented into the scheduling system. Every case should be booked on the basis of the new urgency classification. The surgeon rather than the OR scheduling staff should assign urgency, even though scheduling staff are typically well qualified to make the judgment. The new system depends on surgeon participation and compliance, so it is important that the surgeon decide the urgency. In addition, it is important that urgency be determined at the time of booking and not later. Similarly, urgency should not be modified after the case is booked except in instances in which patient condition has changed. Implementing this new urgency classification is the first key step toward separating nonelective flows that are randomly occurring from work-ins and truly elective cases, which can be managed to optimize hospital flow.

Separating Nonelective Flow. When randomly occurring unscheduled cases can be reliably identified, we can use queuing methodology to determine the resources needed to accommodate them with quality and efficiency. The first step is to prepare the data (arrival rate and average case length) needed for queuing analysis. Each arrival pattern for each urgency subgrouping of unscheduled cases should be tested for randomness. If there is no artificial variability present, the arrival pattern normally follows

a Poisson distribution.

Artificial variability in urgent/emergent arrivals may be present for a variety of reasons (for example, patients being directed by their primary care physicians [PCPs] to go to a hospital ED during off hours or vacation days when the PCP group has inadequate coverage). Such a practice results in arrival times that do not follow a statistically random pattern. Artificial variability might also occur when arrivals are transferred from other hospitals or physicians' offices (based on the physicians' convenience) or when surgeons batch scheduled and unscheduled cases together before presenting them to the scheduling office for OR time. Because queuing models appropriate for this application assume a Poisson distribution (*see* Chapter 5) for arrivals, it is critical to eliminate any artificial variability to ensure accurate results. Otherwise, inappropriate modeling could significantly overstate needed resources, producing waste, or understating needed resources, thereby jeopardizing access.

After arrival patterns have been examined to calculate arrival rates, average case length should be calculated as time from patient-in-the-OR to out-of-OR plus room turnaround time (from patient out of room to room ready for next patient). This information should be fed into a multiserver, multipriority queuing model to determine the resources needed for the nonelective flows. Queuing analysis provides information on the trade-off between resource levels (number of staffed ORs) and expected waiting times for the different nonelective urgency classes. As the number of rooms is increased, expected waiting times decrease, but so does expected room utilization. *An acceptable model is one where projected average waiting times are well within the limits stipulated*

Table 4-1. Two Hospitals' Urgency Groupings

Hospital A	Hospital B
A: 30 minutes	A: 30 minutes
B: 2 hours	B: 4 hours
C: 4 hours	C: 12 hours
D: 8 hours	D: 24 hours
E: 24 hours	E: Work-ins, select procedures, 1–3 days
F: Inpatient work-ins, 1–5 days	F: All other elective
G: Elective, 5+ days	

Sources: Palmetto Health Richland, Columbia, South Carolina (Hospital A), and Cincinnati Children's Hospital Medical Center (*see* Chapter 6). Used with permission.

by the urgency classification but not so low that projected room utilization is unacceptably low. For example, queuing analysis might show that two ORs will have an average expected waiting time of 8 minutes for emergencies that need to get in the OR within 30 minutes of booking, while adding another OR might decrease the expected waiting time for these cases to 2 minutes. What is acceptable is entirely up to individual hospitals, but the second scenario is likely to overresource the nonelective flows. Regardless of the number of rooms decided on, overflow plans should be in place for very-low-probability events when multiple emergencies arrive simultaneously. In some instances, a hospital might have a very small proportion (< 5%) of nonelective demand, in which case it may be excessive to set aside even one OR for these flows. Adding semielective cases (work-ins) to the use of this room to increase utilization may be appropriate if the incidence of very urgent cases is low enough, or it may be better to continue to use a bump-and-delay mechanism to accommodate the rare nonelective case.

After a queuing scenario is accepted, in the second step, separate OR resources need to be set aside for the nonelective flows. OR resources include the room(s), equipment, OR staff, anesthesia, and surgeons. Surgeon availability is often the linchpin in making this model work. Surgeons must make themselves available according to the urgency classification system (with specification of wait times) that they developed. Queuing analysis assumes that cases are done solely on the basis of clinical urgency, as soon as resources are available. If this underlying assumption is violated by introducing nonclinically driven delays and modifications, it will not be possible to ensure that urgent/emergent cases will be performed within the clinically acceptable waiting times predicted by the queuing model. Although we have singled out surgeons, the same responsibilities apply to providing anesthesia, nursing, equipment, radiology, and so on, when the OR becomes available.

Separating Work-in Flow. Work-in cases are those that can wait more than 24 hours but need to be performed within a few days. As is the case with nonelective flow, separate capacity and resources need to be devoted to work-in cases if their volume is sufficient. The main challenge for this category is to define the cases that belong in this group. Inpatients are good candidates to include because the effects of a delay in accessing the OR or a catheterization laboratory are a prolonged hospital LOS and potential deterioration in patient condition. Certain morning admission and outpatient procedures may also need to be included—for example, breast biopsy, where both diagnostic and social urgencies play a role in determining acceptable waiting time. Utilization of resources for these semielective cases should be higher than the utilization in the unscheduled area but somewhat lower than block time and rooms devoted to strictly elective cases. Over- or underestimating the volume of this flow leads to waste on the one hand and longer-than-desired waits on the other.

After work-in demand has been determined and assuming that this demand is patient (versus surgeon availability) driven, queuing models can be used to determine capacity based on volume and acceptable maximum waiting times. Alternately, given the nonurgent nature of work-ins, it might be wise to semielectively schedule these cases. If an individual surgeon's or service's flow is small, it makes sense to provide common access. The lower level of urgency allows for more flexibility in scheduling cases on a particular day. Whereas nonelective cases require that providers and staff and all resources be available as soon as the OR is available, work-in cases can be fit into a surgeon's day by "flipping" a surgeon to the work-in room in between elective cases or performing work-ins at the end of the prime-time elective day. Regardless of the method used to accommodate work-ins, separating them from the elective schedule allows for higher utilization of elective block time, which increases overall utilization and efficiency in the OR.

Conducting Compliance Review. To ensure that all constituents do their part to comply with the urgency classification, a system of checks and balances needs to be established. A compliance process typically involves periodic review of all cases falling outside established criteria for waiting times (that is, a case exceeded the stipulated waiting time) or those with evidence of manipulation of the urgency code. Review is performed either by an authorized person (typically the OR director or surgical medical director) or an administrative body such as an OR committee. Surgeons may "game" the urgency coding system to manipulate OR access. For example, a surgeon might "upcode" a case to get an OR immediately, even if the clinical condition does not warrant it. Take the example of a procedure that needs to get done within 12 hours from booking, according to a surgeon's original urgency classification. Let's say the case occurs on a Friday, when the surgeon has social plans for the evening. Instead of handing that case to a partner, the surgeon wants to do it himself, so at the time of scheduling, he classifies that patient as a four-hour case to ensure that he gets access to the unscheduled OR. This might jeopardize OR access for a truly emergent patient with a higher urgency priority. A longer-term consequence of upcoding is that if the proportion of more urgent cases goes up, more OR resources will need to be devoted to these flows, at the cost of resources for the purely elective flows. Similarly, downcoding may provide a surgeon the ability to delay urgent cases until after office hours (or whatever other activity is being given preference), potentially at the risk of causing harm to the patient. In the longer term, downcoding could lead to decreased resources for urgent flows and increased resources for elective flows. The elective blocks would then not be fully utilized because of a need to provide time to accommodate more unscheduled or work-in cases inappropriately coded as elective but not capable of waiting longer periods of time. Given the negative quality-of-care implications for noncompliance with urgency classification, semipublic review with some peer pressure is often sufficient, but on occasion, it may be necessary to invoke the power of a medical executive or hospitalwide quality committee to change behavior.[21]

Reallocating Elective Prime Time and Separating Day-Surgery Flows. Aside from ensuring timely access for nonelective and work-in cases, the main reason for separating those cases from electively scheduled cases is that it permits maximum efficiency and increases elective throughput. Again, as discussed previously, separating homogenous groups is an essential principle for increasing performance in this electively scheduled group of patients—in this case by optimally managing natural clinical variability. (For an unscheduled group of patients, such as ED patients, the same principle holds, as seen in the frequent separation of fast-track patients from those requiring more extensive diagnostic and treatment services.)

The first separation to be made is to distinguish patients going home the same day (outpatients) from patients being admitted to inpatient floors after surgery (morning admissions). Day-surgery cases are different, not just because those patients are expected to go home after the procedure but also because of differences in the preoperative and recovery processes and the types of anesthesia techniques used. Moreover, the room setup and turnaround process is much shorter than for the more complex inpatient cases. Mixing day-surgery and inpatient cases can lengthen the preoperative, recovery, and room turnaround for the day-surgery cases—which in turn reduces the overall potential throughput for the OR—than if the day-surgery cases follow one after the other, hence the need to separate day surgery blocks from morning admission blocks. OR capacity needed for day-surgery is calculated separately from inpatient demand on the basis of volume of cases (it is important not to double-count nonelective and work-in cases in either group) and average case length (including turnover time), assuming 100% scheduling efficiency:

Number of Scheduled Cases × Average Case Length (Including Turnover) Divided by Efficiency

For example, if a service does 20 cases per month, and the average case length, including turnover time, is 150 minutes, that service's total block time per month should be 3,000 minutes.

Blocks can then be provided to individuals or groups of surgeons if their volume justifies, or to the service in general. Although block time is allocated on the basis of 100% scheduling efficiency,

a somewhat lower actual utilization should be expected because of cancellations, delays, and unexpected changes in case length. Because the elective schedule is not going to be disrupted by randomly occurring nonelective cases or semielective work-ins, actual block prime-time utilization of at least 90% is achievable.

Even if all OR prime time is currently blocked for surgeons or services and there are no obvious rooms to designate as unscheduled or work-in, once the unscheduled and work-in cases are stripped out of the elective schedule, prime time will be available to be reallocated for these flows. In some instances, this may require substantial movement of surgeons or services to different days or times of day for their blocks. In this case, it may be worthwhile to consider simultaneous design and implementation of Phase 2 (Smoothing Elective Flows), which may also require movement of surgical blocks.

Phase 1 Benefits. A list of potential benefits for every hospital as a direct result of Phase 1 implementation includes the following:

- Decreased wait times for urgent/emergent cases, thereby improving clinical outcomes as well as decreasing LOS and improving patient flow
- Increased effective capacity for surgical and cardiac catheterization growth without addition of commensurate resources
- Decreased overtime as more cases are handled during prime time
- Decreased cancellation or delay of elective surgeries to accommodate higher-urgency cases
- Improved patient, provider, and staff satisfaction

For example, Palmetto Health Richland Hospital (Columbia, SC) saw a 38% decrease in waiting time for nonelective cases and an $8 million annual margin growth opportunity after implementing Phase 1.[22] The free ROI Estimator calculator is available on the Institute for Healthcare Optimization Web site* for any hospital to calculate an individualized estimate of increase in throughput and financial benefit from Phase 1. Phase 1 can be applied in settings other than the OR—that is, wherever random and scheduled demands are mixed. The benefits resulting from improved efficiency and better alignment between demand and capacity, thereby optimizing patient flow, are similar to those described.

Phase 2: Smoothing Elective Flows

Phase 1 serves as an important building block in improving overall

---

* The institute can be contacted at http://www.ihoptimize.org/methodology.htm, and access to the calculator is granted on request.

hospital flow. Its benefits accrue mainly to the OR and the catheterization laboratory, with positive effects on flow in the rest of the hospital, particularly in terms of access for urgent/emergent patients and patient flow to inpatient units. In Phase 1, the benefits are targeted directly at downstream (for example, inpatient units) and upstream (ED) areas. The goal of Phase 2 is to eliminate or at least minimize the negative effects on inpatient units of variability in elective inpatient bed demand. These effects are easily identified as wide swings in the number of admissions from day to day, coupled with wide swings in inpatient unit census. The unfortunate combination of a peak in admission demand and a full unit causes patients to be delayed or inappropriately placed, and it may lead to an increase in medical errors due to an acute decrease in nurse-to-patient staffing.

Establishing Admission and Discharge Criteria.
Establishing the urgency classification, as described in "Phase 1: Homogenization and Separation of Elective and Nonelective Flows," clearly distinguishes the different types of demands (elective, work-in, urgent/emergent) for hospital inpatient beds. In addition to classifying the type of demand, it is important to establish clear admission and discharge criteria for every inpatient unit. Doing so creates the foundation for a design to ensure appropriate patient placement as well as clinically appropriate LOS on every unit. Admission criteria are typically based on a combination of patient characteristics (for example, age), clinical service (surgical procedure), care needs (ventilator, presence of lines), and the unit's care capabilities. Discharge criteria are typically based on the patient's care progression and care needs. All admitting physicians must agree and adhere to the criteria, with compliance review similar to the urgency review in the OR for unscheduled and work-in cases, as described earlier. The inpatient placement algorithm should include both a standardized preferred and alternative acceptable destination for every patient. Then it becomes possible to associate a preferred destination unit with each elective surgical patient, thereby establishing the demand pattern (that is, admission rate) for every unit.

Admission rate, however, is only one factor to take into account in developing an optimally smoothed design; the other key factor is LOS in the preferred destination unit. The total daily demand for inpatient beds is calculated as follows:

> Number of Admissions × Average LOS = Average Demand for Inpatient Beds
>
> *For example, if the number of admissions per day is 3 and the average LOS on the unit is 2 days, then the average number of beds needed is 3 × 2 = 6 beds. Note that the distribution of LOS will affect how many beds are needed on a daily basis and will vary around the average of 6 beds.*

This is where discharge criteria become very important. Ordinarily, one would assume that patient LOS is only naturally variable, driven by a patient's recovery process, and cannot be modified. Unfortunately, dysfunctional management of the discharge process frequently introduces artificial variability in LOS. The absence or weakness of specific discharge criteria makes it unclear when specific patients should expect to be discharged from a particular unit. Even if discharge readiness is known, patients may not be discharged when they are ready because of downstream bottlenecks—for example, at another unit in the hospital, at another facility (such as a rehabilitation facility), or due to delayed escorts. Whether or not discharge destination is an issue, dysfunctional discharge processes may unnecessarily increase LOS. For example, a unit may have a practice of working on discharges only after a number of other daily activities are completed, thus delaying the discharge sometimes to the next day. The end result is that the recorded LOS for patients of a particular unit cannot be assumed to be exponentially distributed, as would be expected if the LOS were only naturally variable. *It is as important to identify and eliminate artificial variability in discharge flow as it is important to prevent it in the demand for admissions.* If LOS appears clinically driven and can be accurately measured, the final step to prepare for a design is to determine whether there are homogeneous groups of patients with similar LOS in the demand for each unit. Smoothing the admission demand for each LOS subgroup separately will result in optimal design to reduce variability in census and workload.

Determining Smoothing Priority

In deciding on an elective surgery smoothing approach to optimize unit function, it is important to consider separately the two major determinants of workload and stress on the inpatient units: the day-to-day variability in the number of elective admissions to the unit and the day-to-day variability in overall census.

• *Variability in Elective Admissions.* Because much of the critical nursing workload occurs during the first 24 hours of admission, the number of admissions per day can be a major source of stress, somewhat independent of a unit's census. The biggest source of artificial variability in admissions to inpatient units is the weekend/holiday phenomenon. Most hospitals admit minimal to no elective patients on Saturdays, Sundays, and hospital holidays. This in and of itself reduces both census and daily work intensity during weekends and holidays and underutilizes bed capacity during the weekends. The only truly optimal and maximally smoothed admission pattern is to spread the same number of elective admissions, by preferred destination unit, in each LOS homogeneous subgroup equally across all days of the week. This would produce both the same number of admissions per day and a steady census each day within the bounds of clinical variability in LOS. Capacity could then be appropriately established so that patient flow is optimally managed. Because seven-day-a-week elective surgery (or catheterization laboratory and other elective admissions) is not currently available at most hospitals, an intuitive next-best solution might be to perform the same number of surgeries each weekday on patients in each LOS subgroup. However, before deciding on this smoothing design, let us consider in more detail the second determinant of unit workload—the daily census.

• *Variability in Daily Census.* What is it we care most about for the units—the daily number of admissions and discharges, the census level, or both? Both are determinants of daily nursing workload. Although nurse staffing level is often described in terms of nurse-to-patient (census) ratios, the impact of admissions, transfers, and discharges on nursing workload is not insignificant. Any Phase 2 design should attempt to smooth both inpatient admissions and census simultaneously (which is possible when elective surgeries are performed seven days a week). Unfortunately, this is impossible to achieve if one performs elective surgery only five days a week. Doing the same number of elective surgeries that require inpatient admission each weekday could result, depending on LOS, in a census increasing during the first few days of the week to a peak on Thursday or Friday, then declining to a minimum on Monday morning. It is possible to create a design, using simulation modeling, to minimize the weekly increase in census by admitting different numbers of patients in each homogenous LOS subgroup while at the same time producing as smooth an admission pattern across all days of the week. If the priority for the hospital is to achieve a maximally smooth weekday census, then the OR may have to tolerate and plan for predictable differences in surgical caseload for some services on regular weekdays.

Census level, apart from being a determinant of nurse-to-patient staffing levels, is also a key driver of overall hospital throughput. *A consistently high hospital occupancy maximizing utilization of inpatient beds without serious bottlenecks and increased LOS can occur only if minimal fluctuations in day-to-day census are allowed.* If the overall goal of Phase 2 is to better utilize hospital beds while at the same time maintaining quality of care, then smoothing census should take priority over smoothing daily inpatient admissions. After the final design priority for smoothing unit census versus admission rate is decided, simulation modeling should be used to determine the optimal number of elective surgeries to be performed each working day for patients in each LOS subgroup of procedures for each preferred destination. Again, a seven-day surgical schedule would allow a hospital to simultaneously (1) significantly increase patient throughput and maximally utilize

hospital resources, (2) smooth hospital census, and (3) smooth elective admissions to the units, thereby optimally managing patient flow. We do recognize that doing so would introduce a significant change in hospital practices, which requires carefully considered implementation, as we now discuss.

Implementing a New Surgery Schedule. A new schedule for elective surgery is implemented using two complementary maneuvers. The first is to move the block days of select providers to achieve the average desired number of admissions to each unit for each day of the week, as indicated by the simulation modeling. For example, when smoothing the orthopedic inpatient unit, the design might indicate that an average of eight procedures are to be performed each Monday. This may be possible to accomplish via a particular combination of orthopedic surgeons on Mondays. This block reallocation will produce an OR schedule that smoothes the daily schedule on average, but some peaks and valleys may still remain from case-mix variability on any given day. This remaining variability is minimized using a second maneuver—a system of caps (maximum number of cases that can be scheduled) on the number of specific LOS subgroup cases to be performed on any given day. For example, if the design calls for six total joints to be done on Mondays, a cap of six cases per day would prevent any given Monday from overloading the orthopedic inpatient unit. Cases displaced by a cap on any given day will fill in the valleys on another day, thus causing the actual caseload to come as close as possible to the design. When caps are high enough to accommodate average load and then some, there is no restriction on any service or surgeon case volume.

When smoothing the flows to numerous units across many services, substantial reallocation and movement of elective blocks may be necessary. If reallocation is needed in Phase 1 to provide dedicated unscheduled and work-in rooms, it may be useful to implement Phases 1 and 2 together to produce one new block design rather than experience two major block changes sequentially. The end result of Phase 2 implementation is a new OR schedule and block reallocation for elective surgery that produces a smoothed demand from the OR for inpatient beds to achieve a high, minimally variable floor census, maximal utilization of floor beds, and optimal management of patient flow.

Phase 2 Benefits. Phase 2 benefits include the following:

■ Increased use of inpatient capacity for growth without addition of commensurate resources
■ Improved patient placement in appropriate units, thereby improving quality of care
■ Decreased waiting times for elective patients to get in to appropriate units, resulting in improved patient flow
■ Decreased variability and increased predictability in nursing

workload and decreased stress on nurses
- Decreased variability in nurse-to-patient staffing ratios
- Decreased ED boarding and increased ED throughput as a result of decreased competition from elective admissions, thereby improving patient flow
- Improved patient, provider, and staff satisfaction

Phase 2 smoothing can be applied wherever there is a large schedulable or elective flow (for example, catheterization laboratory, endoscopy, certain areas of radiology) and will result in benefits similar to those listed for OR smoothing.

Phase 3: Estimation of Resource Needs

Under conditions of optimally managed patient flow, a hospital can confidently determine the resources (or capacity) needed to serve a given patient demand for services. Before implementing Phases 1 and 2, it would not be possible to answer the oft-asked question "How many beds do we need in unit X?" When artificial variability causes unpredictable, nonrandom peaks and valleys in demand, there can be no accurate answer to this question. However, once the smoothing process of Phase 2 has been implemented and the remaining variability in census reflects clinically driven variability in LOS and random changes in demand from urgent/emergent patients, it is possible to determine unit capacity within a narrow range.

Capacity needs are determined separately for each patient flow to the unit. The number of beds needed for randomly arriving patients—that is, from the ED—is determined using queuing models, which show the bed capacity needed to accommodate most new patient arrivals within specified maximum waiting times. Sensitivity analyses can be performed to show the trade-offs between bed occupancy rates on the one hand and mean waiting times and the percentage of patients whose waits will exceed the accepted standard on the other. An important consideration is that the queuing models appropriate for such health care applications assume random Poisson arrivals and exponential LOS, which means that LOS is assumed to be purely clinically determined. Before queuing analyses are performed, the data should be checked for both of these assumptions. If LOS is not exponentially distributed, then the source of artificial variability (for example, patient boarding time) needs to be determined and extracted from the overall LOS. As discussed earlier, the discharge timing and process often contributes to artificial variability. Discharges are delayed for social and administrative reasons, such as late rounding and delays in orders, laboratory tests, transfer of patients to postacute facilities, and so on.

The number of beds needed for elective arrivals is determined

using simulation modeling.[4] The simulation model in Phase 2 can easily be extended to determine the number of beds that will be needed for the smoothed schedule. The number of beds is determined on the basis of a particular hospital's tolerance for overflow to a secondary unit. For example, if zero overflow to a less desirable postsurgical unit is acceptable, the number of beds needed would increase because of the natural variability in LOS. If, say, 5% overflow is acceptable, the model would provide exactly the number of beds that would be sufficient 95% of the time. The overflow targets are set using hospital and provider comfort level with accommodating these patients in alternate units some of the time. These same methods can be used for planning purposes to determine the number of beds that would be needed for anticipated growth in a particular service line. With the capital cost of a new inpatient bed estimated at $1 million and an annual operating expense per bed in excess of $250,000,[23] knowing exactly the number of beds (or other similarly costly health care assets, such as ORs and radiology) needed to provide quality care has substantial financial implications.

Phase 3 Benefits. Phase 3 benefits include the following:
- Decreased patient misplacement, resulting in higher quality of care and potentially lower LOS
- Decreased interunit transfers, often resulting in shorter LOS and improved patient flow
- Improved nursing satisfaction
- Objective ability to adjust bed assignments to accommodate changes in demand, thereby more consistently and reliably aligning capacity with changing demand to ensure optimal patient flow
- Decreased ED boarding times and frequency, thereby reducing LOS and improving patient flow
- Avoidance of the cost of building and staffing unnecessary unit beds

These benefits accrue to inpatient units, and similar benefits can be achieved by rightsizing procedural areas such as laboratories and radiology.

Implementation Considerations

While there is nothing sacrosanct about the order in which the various parts of Phases 1 and 2 are undertaken, the three-phase sequencing takes into account typical data availability, the ability of an organization to adopt change, and the ability to reap early benefits to ensure stakeholder engagement. Generally, Phase 1 should precede Phase 2 because it is difficult to smooth elective OR or catheterization laboratory flows when they are constantly interrupted by nonelective demands. As described in Chapter 3, an overall patient flow assessment can provide key insights into a particular hospital's bottleneck points. Sometimes a hospital may have very clear and significant bottlenecks in particular areas that may warrant modifying the sequencing of the various recommended phases. For example, if a particular inpatient unit is constantly overloaded and rejecting patients (as opposed to doing so only on certain days), it may be necessary to add a few beds to that unit sooner rather than later. The challenge is in determining how many beds are needed for elective admissions when smoothing has not been done. A very rough approach is to look at historical census data for a particular unit and then estimate bed needs on the basis of various scenarios of overflow to alternative units. For example, if a maximum 10% overflow to other units is acceptable, you need more beds than if a 20% overflow is acceptable. Although likely not accurate (because artificial variability might cause the future patterns to differ from the historical ones), this calculation would provide a range of estimates of beds needed. This number of beds would still be inadequate, with artificial variability left unaddressed, but it could help alleviate acute bed needs without adding excessive resources. In such a scenario, it would also be appropriate to combine Phases 1 and 2 by undertaking smoothing of elective flow earlier in the process to relieve the stress of artificial variability on the inpatient units.

The main goal of a redesign is to optimally manage patient flow and increase throughput in the system without imposing delays or reducing quality of care. The end result is that more capacity for new demand becomes available after the first two phases. For a hospital implementing this redesign, greater efficiency and reduced waits can act as magnets for attracting new patients and providers. However, if the current variability or excess capacity is very high relative to the growth opportunity for a particular hospital, it may not be possible to fill the freed-up capacity. In this case, the only option would be to close ORs or unit beds.

Political realities often play a significant role in the day-to-day execution of the redesign. It is important to understand the effects of the new design and policies on various constituents. For example, surgeons may be required to change how they schedule and when they perform certain types of cases. This change in practice may require changes in their other work flows—clinical, teaching, or administrative. Department meetings and tumor boards are frequent examples of conflicts with on-time starts in the OR. Similarly, changes to OR and anesthesia staffing and shifts may become necessary; for example, unscheduled ORs are typically staffed using generalist teams, which may make some surgeons uncomfortable with the change. Exceptions may need to be made, but they are best made sparingly and strategically so that the overall design fundamentals are not violated. One useful tactic is to make exceptions on a time-limited basis and phase them out

gradually. A hospital–physician partnership approach may elongate the time it takes to implement but has incredible value in delivering a sustainable design.

A find but quite important consideration is leadership commitment and the investment in project management and data analysis expertise. The success of such a major patient flow redesign initiative is predicated on consistent leadership support from the board on down. It is also extremely useful to identify and empower a few key physician champions for patient flow improvement. Finally, project management and data analysis constitute the greatest demand on personnel effort. These staff play a key role in ensuring continuous forward momentum and analytic rigor in the process.

Other Tools for Patient Flow Management

Although VM, as implemented in the three-phase approach described earlier, is designated as a tool for managing organizational variability (as recommended by the American Hospital Association[24]), a number of additional and complementary approaches to patient flow improvement need to be considered. These approaches can generally be described as process improvement methodologies. A few of the most important ones are now described, along with recommendations on how to incorporate these tools into patient flow improvement strategies.

Bed/Capacity Management

Dynamic bed management systems play an important role in providing near-term visibility into bed needs and bed availability. A bed management system can be used as a platform to improve communication across teams to facilitate smoother movement of patients across the continuum of care. For example, bed management can be powerful in improving timely discharges, thereby reducing LOS and reducing ED and PACU holds typical during the middle of the day. Reducing delays and service time (LOS) decreases artificial variability and improves patient flow. Many hospitals use bed management programs as early warning systems to identify emerging bottlenecks, that may affect new admissions. They then work to quickly identify free beds and to expedite turnaround. Some of these systems offer discharge planning that can help hospitals obtain a higher level of control over patient flow.

Bed management systems can also incorporate LOS predictions, particularly for elective admissions that may be helpful in predicting future system overloads.[25] It is too soon to say whether this information can be accurate enough across a wide range of services to warrant modification of future admission demand. A key distinction between variability and bed management methodologies is that dynamic bed management is an attempt to manage chaos, whereas VM changes hospital operations to prevent chaos. Bed management systems alone have been shown to improve patient throughput and utilization of hospital beds.[26] However, applying VM first would greatly enhance the benefits of dynamic day-to-day management of patient flows. Finally, bed management systems complement VM by providing a means to continuously measure (for example, percentage of patients placed in first preferred unit, waiting time to get into a unit) and improve patient flow performance.

Radio Frequency Identification/Patient Tracking

In addition to bed management, patient tracking is another dynamic flow management tool, except that it centers on the patient instead of beds. Hospitals have used patient tracking to improve handoffs and reduce delays in the patient journey.[27,28] A patient tracking system can facilitate the entry of time stamps that are not currently captured, such as a patient being ready for next step of care process. Such data are very useful for the three-phase Redesign of Patient Flow Management approach. Such a system can also be integrated into an active compliance process by flagging patients whose waiting time is approaching stipulated maximums.

Similar to bed management systems, radio frequency identification (RFID) systems can help expose bottlenecks in a real-time manner and enable quick management interventions, but they do not address the root causes of patient flow issues facing hospitals. Yet RFID, like dynamic bed management, can serve as a powerful continuous improvement complement to VM.

Risks of Applying Process Improvement Methodologies Incorrectly

Applying process improvement tools, such as the ones just described, before addressing artificial variability will likely produce some flow improvement, but the results might be diminished or even negated by unaddressed inherent variability. For example, improving communication and coordination across departments should improve patient flow, but even the best communication process will fail in the face of excessive fluctuations in nurse-to-patient staffing ratios caused by artificial variability (*see* the OR turnover example, page 48). At worst, process improvement before process redesign could result in further entrenchment of bad practices, making the redesign work even more difficult.

Another risk of process improvement without regard for structural design is that it ignores key operations management principles such as the distinction between elective and random arrivals. Resources for elective patients can be programmed for nearly 100% efficiency, while random arrivals require a lower utilization to ensure timely access. The relationship between resource needs for random arrivals and waiting times can be explored only with the help of queuing models. If waste reduction through Lean management eliminates all or most of the flexibility in a system, the result would be unacceptable delays for urgent patients and compromised quality of care. The bottom line is that process improvement methods should follow structural design improvements to maximize the benefit for hospitalwide patient flow.

Summary and Conclusions

Patient flow management plays a crucial role in health care delivery, not only in terms of quality and patient safety but, as seen more recently, in costs and revenue. Many different approaches to patient flow management are available, and some have shown promising results. In this chapter we focus on OM and VM as necessary foundations for patient flow management. OM methodologies such as queuing models and simulation have been successfully applied in several industries to reduce cost and improve service and quality. However, these standard OM tools cannot be applied to health care without addressing the core problem of artificial variability. Artificial variability is a result of inappropriate management, as compared with natural variability, which is an artifact of patients' clinical needs. From the perspective of hospital patient flow, artificial variability in scheduled admissions—elective surgical and cardiac procedures and certain scheduled medical admissions (mostly in cancer services)—is the main source of significant systemwide problems. The presence of artificial variability in health care decreases access to services, increases chaos and staff stress, decreases patient safety and quality of care, decreases staff and patient satisfaction, increases cost, and decreases overall system throughput. The common problem of ED overcrowding represents perhaps the most visible effect of artificial variability. It has been established that a significant cause of ED overcrowding is the flow of scheduled admissions.

We presented a three-phase VM-based process for patient flow redesign, which entails separating scheduled and unscheduled flows, smoothing the flow (that is, eliminating artificial variability) of scheduled patients, and determining resources using OM tools such as queuing and simulation models. After implementing the VM-based three-step patient flow redesign process, other improvement approaches, such as bed management and patient tracking, can be employed to further enhance patient flow.

In summary, the key principles of a patient flow management strategy are that it should have a systemwide perspective, it should be science based and data driven, it should provide the right structure, and it should include a systematic compliance review and enforcement process.

The authors extend special thanks to Kathleen Fuda, Ph.D., and Adam Rutenberg, M.B.A., for their assistance and comments.

References

1. Litvak E.: Optimizing patient flow by managing its variability. In *Front Office to Front Line: Essential Issues for Health Care Leaders.* Oakbrook Terrace, IL : Joint Commission Resources, 2005, pp. 91–111.

2. Carter M., Price C.: *Operations Research: A Practical Introduction.* Boca Raton, FL: CRC Press LLC, 2001.

3. Hillier F.S., Lieberman G.J.: *Queuing Theory: Introduction to Operations Research.* New York: McGraw-Hill, 2005.

4. Kuljis J., Paul R.J., Stergioulas L.K.: *Can Health Care Benefit from Modeling and Simulation Methods in the Same Way as Business and Manufacturing Has?* Piscataway, NJ : IEEE Press, 2007. Proceedings of the 2007 Winter Simulation Conference, pp. 1449–1453.

5. Vissers J., Beech R.: *Health Operations Management: Patient Flow Logistics in Health Care.* Saddle River, NJ: Routledge Health Management Services, 2005.

6. Litvak E., Long M.: Cost and quality under managed care: Irreconcilable differences? *Am J Manag Care* 6:305–312, Mar. 2000.

7. Program for Management of Variability in Health Care Delivery: *Improving Patient Flow and Throughput in California Hospitals Operating Room Services.* Prepared for the California Healthcare Foundation, 2007, Chapters 5 and 6. http://www.bu.edu/mvp/Library/CHCF%20Guidance%20document.pdf (accessed Jul. 14, 2009).

8. McManus M.L., et al.: Variability in demand and access to pediatric intensive care services. *Anesthesiology* 98:1491–1496, Jun. 2003.

9. Aiken H., et al.: Hospital nurse staffing and patient mortality, nurse burnout, and job dissatisfaction. *JAMA* 288:1987–1993, Oct. 23–30, 2002.

10. Litvak E, et al.: Managing unnecessary variability in patient demand to reduce nursing stress and improve patient safety. *Jt Comm J Qual Patient Saf* 31:330–338, Jun. 2005.

11. Richardson D.B.: The access-block effect: Relationship between delay to reaching an inpatient bed and inpatient length of stay. *Med J Aust* 177:492–495, Nov. 4, 2002.

12. Novack V., et al.: Does delay in surgery after hip fracture lead to worse outcomes? A multicenter survey. *Int J Qual Health Care* 19:170–176, Jun. 2007.

13. Bastani A., Anderson W., Spiro O.: How long before patients lose their patience? *Ann Emerg Med* 52(Suppl. 1 to issue 4):S86–S87, Oct. 2008.

14. American Hospital Association: *AHA Hospital Statistics.* Chicago: Health Forum, 2009.

15. Institute of Medicine: *Hospital-Based Emergency Care: At the Breaking Point.* Washington, DC: National Academies Press, 2006.

16. U.S. General Accountability Office (GAO): *Hospital Emergency Departments: Crowding Continues to Occur, and Some Patients Wait Longer Than Recommended Time Frames,* Apr. 2009. http://www.gao.gov/new.items/d09347.pdf (accessed Jul. 15, 2009).

17. Carpenter D.: Boom going bust? Credit and financial crisis make for uncertain hospital construction outlook. *Health Facilities Management Magazine.* Feb. 2009. http://www.hfmmagazine.com/hfmmagazine_app/jsp/articledisplay.jsp?dcrpath=HFMMAGAZINE/Article/data/02FEB2009/0902HFM_FEA_C overStory&domain=HFMMAGAZINE (accessed Jul. 17, 2009).

18. Litvak E., et al.: Emergency department diversion: Causes and solutions. *Acad Emerg Med* 8:1108–1110, Nov. 2001.

19. Litvak E., Cooper A., McManus M.: *Root Cause Analysis of Emergency Department Crowding and Ambulance Diversion in Massachusetts.* Boston: Massachusetts Department of Public Health, Oct. 2002. http://www.mass.gov/Eeohhs2/docs/dph/quality/healthcare/ad_emergency_dept_analysis.pdf (accessed Jul. 17, 2009).

20. McManus M.L., et al.: Queuing theory accurately models the need for critical care resources *Anesthesiology* 100:1271–1276, May 2004.

21. Cosgrove J.F., et al.:Decreasing delays in urgent and expedited surgery in a university teaching hospital through audit and communication between perioperative and surgical directorates. *Anaesthesia* 63:599–603, Jun. 2008.

22. Personal communication between author [S.G.V.] and Ellis M. Knight, M.D., M.B.A., Senior Vice President for Ambulatory Services, Palmetto Health Richland, Columbia, SC, Jun. 30, 2009.

23. Butterfield S.: A new Rx for crowded hospitals: Math. Operations management expert brings queuing theory to healthcare. *ACP Hospitalist,* Dec. 2007. http://www.acphospitalist.org/archives/2007/12/math.htm (accessed Jul. 17, 2009).

24. American Hospital Association: *Hospitals in Pursuit of Excellence.* http://www.ahaqualitycenter.org/qualitycenter/hpoe/content/intro.pdf (accessed Jul. 9, 2009).

25. Van Houdenhoven M.: Optimizing intensive care capacity using individual length-of-stay prediction models. *Crit Care* 11(2):R42, 2007.

26. Howell E.: Active bed management by hospitalists and emergency department throughput. *Ann Intern Med* 149:804–810, Dec. 2, 2008.

27. RFID^SM Solutions Online: *Waco's Providence Health Center Goes Live with Prospective Patient Flow Manager from Radianse,* Mar. 19, 2007. http://www.rfidsolutionsonline.com/article.mvc/Patient-Flow-Manager-Wacos-Providence-Health-0001?VNETCOOKIE=NO (accessed Jul. 17, 2009).

28. Vision™: *A Modern Approach to Quality Care.* http://versustech.com/pdf/WestSound_Success_Story_080306.pdf (accessed Jul. 17, 2009)

Chapter 5

Measurement and Evaluation of Patient Flow: The Right Data, Measures, and Analyses

Kathleen Kerwin Fuda, Ph.D.

This chapter discusses quantitative analysis of patient flow in health care organizations, with a focus on hospitals. Although interviewing relevant staff is a good way to gather initial information about patient flow problems, quantitative analysis is important for the following reasons:

1. Identifying the causes of and solutions to patient flow problems frequently requires examination of the entire organization; crowding or delays in one area may actually be caused by bottlenecks in other steps of the care process. Although most health care staff will be able to identify flow problems and symptoms in their particular unit or department, few, if any, will have the detailed knowledge of the whole system required to identify the source of the problems and to identify what will be required for a solution. Data can precisely measure the extent of the flow problems, pinpoint where they occur, and illuminate the connections among various units and departments.

2. Applications of certain tools developed by operations researchers, which are very valuable for proper management of patient flow, are quantitative in nature; collection of accurate data is critical to their use. These tools, such as queuing models, can provide the basis for informed decision making concerning patient flow improvements.

3. Informative analyses and presentation of an organization's own data can be essential in persuading key staff members of the need for improvements in patient flow and why recommended changes would be beneficial. Because of their scientific training, clinicians often seek clear evidence both of the need for change and how recommended changes would help. Otherwise, natural reluctance to change established patterns of behavior may impede progress on improvements to patient flow patterns.

The Questions Guiding Analysis

Patient flow–related data analyses seek to address the following related questions:

1. Does my hospital have problems with patient flow, and if so, where are they, what are the symptoms, and how serious are they? Analyses to address these questions look at patterns of demand and seek to identify and measure symptoms of patient flow that may be too high or too low for a given capacity for treatment. These may include crowding, delays and waits for services, diversion or rejection of patients presenting for service, substitution of one service for another more suited

to the patient's need, and overtime costs, which are all indicative of at least temporary peaks in demand that overwhelm service capacity. On the other hand, low utilization rates or occupancy rates, excessive staffing ratios and costs, and lower-than-desirable revenues may be symptomatic of at least temporarily low rates of patient demand. Very frequently, both of these types of problems are found within a single hospital because of fluctuating levels of patient demand.

2. What are the causes of the patient flow problems? Although it is commonly assumed that crowding and waits result from inadequate capacity, that may or may not be true. Sometimes improvements in the scheduling of elective admissions, cases, or visits can help to accommodate existing demand within existing capacity; the right measures coupled with the right analyses will identify whether this is possible. Perhaps delays in surgical start times are due to ineffective or inefficient preoperative care processes, lack of identified capacity for urgent cases, late arrivals by surgeons, or patient noncompliance. The solutions will differ depending on the results of your analyses. Perhaps your crowded orthopedic unit has enough beds to meet patients' clinical needs, but difficulties in arranging suitable postacute care are extending patients' length of stay (LOS), blocking admissions of new patients. Perhaps your operating room (OR) is very busy on Mondays, Wednesdays, and Fridays, while your outpatient clinics are swamped on Tuesdays and Thursdays; could there be a connection? Is the wave of emergency department (ED) patients who arrived by ambulance this afternoon merely a chance occurrence, or did the hospital across town go on diversion today?

3. What will be needed to improve patient flow, and what will the trade-offs be? Given existing levels of patient demand, do we have enough beds/treatment rooms/nurses? Do we need to expand capacity to meet tolerable waiting times? Might we comfortably treat additional patients with existing resources? Could we save costs by reducing capacity while still treating all our patients with good quality and acceptable waits? What specific changes do we need to make?

General Data Concerns

Unfortunately, it has only been within the past several years that patient flow has increasingly captured the attention of managers of hospitals and other health care organizations. Health care information systems often reflect this previous lack of interest in that they do not capture certain data useful for monitoring and improving patient flow patterns, or the data collected may be incomplete or of questionable quality. Data problems concerning demand volumes, urgency of care need, and timing of steps in

patient care frequently occur, often reflecting a failure to distinguish between the care that is clinically preferred and the care that is actually provided. Nevertheless, the types of data typically captured in hospitals' information systems, particularly admission, discharge, and transfer (ADT) systems and OR information systems, are generally adequate to carry out many useful analyses. The best approach is to extract the maximum amount of useful information from existing systems while attempting to identify other sources of data. The accuracy and completeness of the data need to be carefully assessed. Data not collected primarily for purposes of patient flow analyses or even used for any reporting purpose may be particularly suspect. Yet *assessment* of patient flow problems (*see* Chapter 3) may not require as rigorous a standard for data accuracy as would analyses carried out to support *implementation* of specific changes in operations, where poor data quality could have more serious consequences.

If there is concern about the accuracy of data, sensitivity analyses may be useful in determining whether the data are sufficiently reliable to support decision making. In sensitivity analysis, a study is conducted to determine how much the analytical outcome changes with changes in the data being analyzed.[1] For example, if overall occupancy rates are relatively high, the estimated waiting time for an ICU bed for emergently admitted patients may change rather dramatically, with small decreases or increases in the average number of admissions or LOS. However, at lower occupancy rates, small differences in arrival rates may not make a substantial difference in waiting times. The more sensitive the calculated outcomes to changes in the data, the more confidence is needed in the accuracy of the data.

Patient Demand

A fundamental goal of patient flow assessment is to describe the demand for patient care of specific types, such as for inpatient stays, ED visits, outpatient surgical procedures, magnetic resonance imaging or computerized tomography scans, or clinic visits, depending on the interests guiding the analysis. It is necessary to determine the volume of demand, when it occurs (date, day of week [DOW], and hour of the day), whether and to what extent it is variable over time, and, if so, why it is variable.

Figure 5-1 (*see* page 77) illustrates the conceptual problems associated with typically available data on demand for specific patient care services, using admissions to two separate inpatient units as an example. Volume statistics can both overestimate and underestimate the demand for specific services by including patients who should not be counted and by excluding patients who should be counted. The figure shows three possible outcomes to patients'

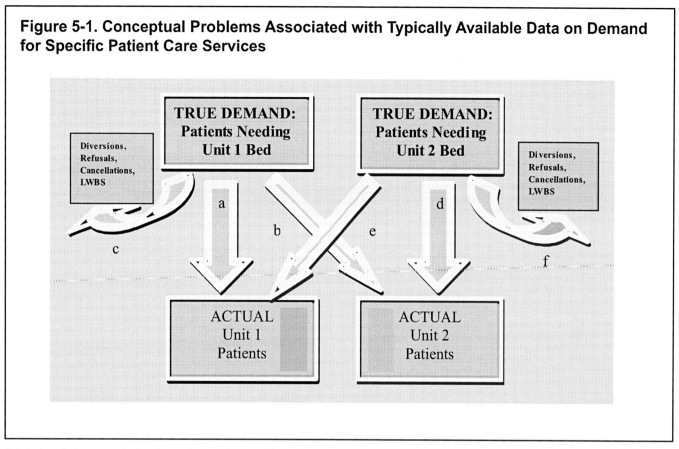

Figure 5-1. Conceptual Problems Associated with Typically Available Data on Demand for Specific Patient Care Services

Admissions to two separate inpatient units are shown to illustrate the conceptual problems associated with typically available data on demand for specific patient care services. The top two boxes indicate the total number of patients requiring care at the hypothetical hospital, divided into two groups on the basis of the type of bed they actually require (according to agreed-on hospital protocols). LWBS, left without being seen.

demand for service. Arrows *a* and *d* indicate patients who received a bed in the unit appropriate for their clinical need (with or without a wait to get in). Arrows *b* and *e* indicate the flows of patients who are provided a bed but in a unit other than the appropriate or optimal one; some patients who would ideally be placed in Unit A are in fact sent to Unit B, and vice versa. Such "off-service" bed placements are a common occurrence in hospitals experiencing periodic crowding; patients are placed in any available bed, as opposed to their optimal bed. Sometimes this may also occur because the admitting physician prefers an "upgraded" level of care, such as a bed in a telemetry unit instead of a regular floor unit, because of the better nursing ratios there or because of some other concern. The result is a mix of patients who are actually placed in beds in each unit, indicated by the boxes at the bottom of the figure: those who "belong" there based on the hospital's standards and those who do not. Finally, arrows *c* and *f* represent the patients who needed treatment but were rejected by the system in some way, so that they had to seek care elsewhere or simply did without care. This flow includes patients such as those transported in diverted ambulances, who do not appear at the hospital where they would otherwise have sought treatment. It also

includes other forms of refusals of treatment, such as refused transfers due to lack of available staffed beds or cancellations due to system problems, as well as patients who abandoned their waits for service and left without being seen (LWBS). This is most commonly recognized as affecting patients seeking treatment in emergency departments (EDs), but the concept is applicable to other sorts of "impatient" patients, such as persons seeking a clinic visit who decide to seek care elsewhere because the first available appointment is too far into the future. In cases of severe crowding, this may sometimes include patients whose condition deteriorates so much during a wait for service that their clinical needs shift to a need for a higher level of care, or they die, or they improve so that they no longer need admission and can go home.

Although we frequently analyze the patterns of *actual* patient placements in a given unit, for other purposes it is preferable to look at *true* demand for the unit (for example, for estimating capacity needs). However, generally the only data easily available to determine the demand for Unit A will be ADT records for the patients who actually stayed there, so that data for the demand represented by arrows *b* and *c* (Figure 5-1) will be missing, thus tending to *under*estimate true demand. Furthermore, the data on actual Unit A patients will include some patients who should have been in Unit B, thus leading to a tendency to *over*restimate demand. The problems in estimating the number of patients who are provided a bed in a nonappropriate or nonoptimal unit (the *b* and *e* flow arrows) are best resolved by establishing clear admissions criteria for each unit (or other relevant service) so that the ideal bed placement for each patient (the "preferred unit") can be recorded, along with the hospital's success in adhering to the criteria monitored. When information systems capture patients' preferred units, data for the misplaced patients in the unit of concern can be excluded from the analysis, while data for the patients who belonged there but were themselves misplaced elsewhere can be added back.

Data issues caused by the *c* and *f* flows tend to be more difficult to fix or to compensate for because detailed data on rejected patients are frequently unavailable. However, sometimes it is possible to make an informed estimate of the number of such rejections. For example, it not usually possible to determine the units to which individual patients subject to ambulance diversion would have been admitted. Instead, an estimate of the average number of patients arriving by ambulance who are admitted by hour to each unit may be applied to the number of hours of diversion each day during the period of analysis. ED data systems will frequently capture some data on LWBS patients, and records may exist for refused interhospital transfers or cancelled admissions or surgical cases, for example. These sorts of data sources can help to compensate or adjust for the underestimate of demand that would otherwise occur.

How much time should the data set cover? In hospitals with significant variation from season to season, analysis of a year's worth of data is ideal to determine what the patterns are. On the other hand, if major changes in operations have recently occurred—for example, opening of new units or ORs—using data from before the change may only confuse the analysis. At a minimum, three months of data is advisable.

Timing Analyses

The first analyses needed are those that describe the volume and timing of demand. Volume needs to be analyzed by date, DOW, and hour of the day. These data, which can pertain to admissions, census, surgical procedures, radiology or clinical laboratory tests, clinic visits, or whatever other service is relevant to the project, can be used to determine both the average level of demand and the extent of its variability. Often it is useful to perform this basic analysis looking at all dates first (*see* Figure 5-2, below) to get a sense of the overall pattern and then to limit the data to nonholiday weekdays (*see* Figure 5-3, page 79) because these are usually the "normal business" times in a hospital or clinic.

The variability of demand can be measured in the following ways:

1. Range of Values. The range of values often represents surprising extremes; the maximum number may be two, three, or even more times the minimum value in the case of admissions, procedures, or visits. Hospital managers are often not fully aware of the range of conditions under which their units or departments are operating nor how often because most existing data reports tend to focus on averages.

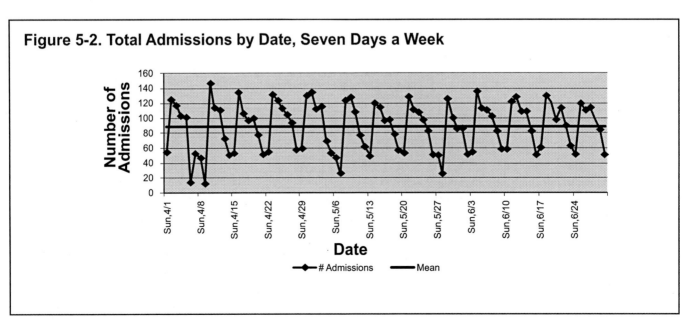

Figure 5-2. Total Admissions by Date, Seven Days a Week

Data are shown for total admissions for 13 consecutive weeks.

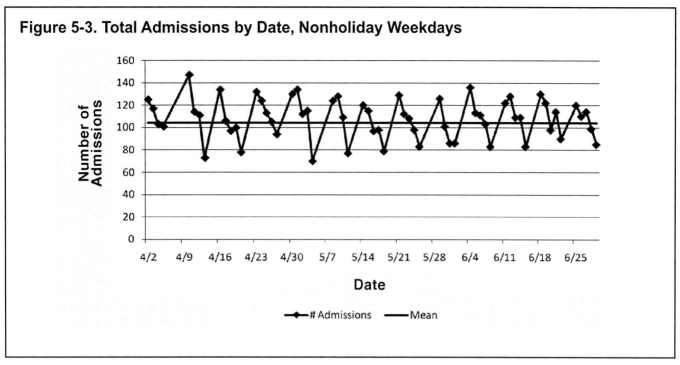

Figure 5-3. Total Admissions by Date, Nonholiday Weekdays

Data are shown for total admissions for 13 consecutive weeks (weekdays).

2. Standard Deviation (S.D.). The S.D. is a frequently used measure of variability, but it should be interpreted cautiously because the distribution of values will not necessarily be normal. Therefore, it cannot be assumed that the usual proportions of values fall within one or two S.D.s of the mean.

3. Coefficient of Variation. The coefficient of variation is useful when the goal is to compare the degree of variability among a number of different units, or services, or clinics. Expressed as a percentage of the mean, it is calculated as follows:

$$S.D./Mean \times 100$$

The higher the percentage, the higher the variability of the values around the mean.

Analyses of DOW patterns can be useful in pointing to potential causes of variability. For example, a census pattern that drops off rapidly on Saturdays and Sundays and then builds to peak late in the workweek (*see* Figure 5-4, page 80) likely reflects low numbers of elective admissions on weekends, and possibly a concentration of discharges on Fridays and Saturdays. Likewise, significant differences in volumes of surgery from one day of the week to another (*see* Figure 5-5, page 80), particularly to a specific unit or by service, often reflects the block schedule and/or uneven allocation of outpatient procedures across the days of the week within surgeons' blocks.

However, it should be remembered that these DOW data, which portray averages, can conceal considerable variability from week to week on any given weekday (*see* Figure 5-6, page 81).

Hour-of-day analyses can illuminate a number of flow problems and their sources. For example, Figure 5-7 (page 81) portrays a hospital unit's mean hourly census across nonholiday weekdays.

Plotting the mean numbers of admissions and discharges per hour can point to the source of similar patterns. For example, for the nursing unit represented in Figure 5-8 (page 82), discharges do not occur smoothly across the day but rather are concentrated in the afternoon and early evening, while admissions occur around the clock, although at higher levels during the day, when elective admissions occur. The potential impact of such a pattern, especially when repeated on multiple units, on flow within the hospital is shown in Figure 5-9 (page 82). The figure shows the mean wait for an inpatient bed by patients ready to leave the PACU. During the late morning, the waits may tend to increase because not enough beds in the nursing units are yet emptied of today's discharges (and readied for the next patient) relative to the number of surgical admissions rapidly emerging from the OR; in the late afternoon, the PACU empties out as beds are freed up and the elective surgery schedule is completed.

Useful analytical breakdowns of time-related analyses may include admissions to each unit, or at least key units at the hospital, especially those where crowding or waits are a concern; sources of demand, such as the OR versus the ED (*see* Figure 5-10, page 83); or activity, by service or individual provider (*see* Figure 5-11, page 83). These may be used for any of the time-related analyses described. Another, often eye-opening, exercise is to look

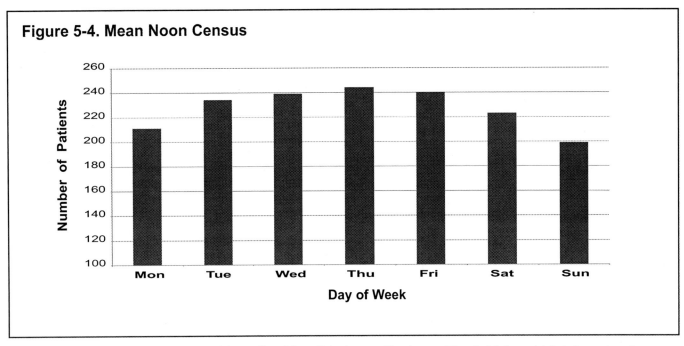

Figure 5-4. Mean Noon Census

As shown in the figure, the mean noon census drops off rapidly on Saturdays and Sundays and then builds to peak late in the workweek.

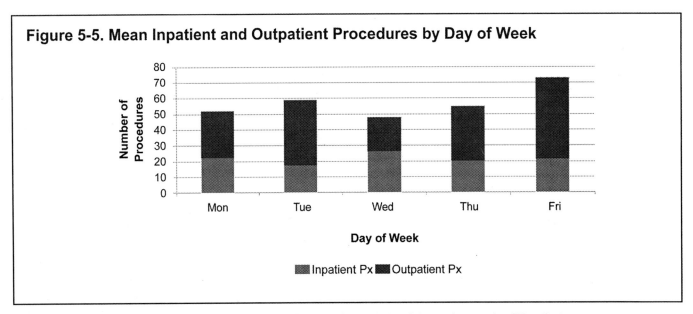

Figure 5-5. Mean Inpatient and Outpatient Procedures by Day of Week

This figure portrays significant differences in mean volumes of surgery from one day of the week to another. PX, patients.

at the variability in patient-to-nurse ratio that is caused by variability in unit census and perhaps in staffing levels. This can be done from date to date, shift to shift, or even hour to hour, if the data are available (*see* Figure 5-12, page 84)

What Is Causing the Variability in Demand over Time?

As described in Chapter 4, the type of variability in demand determines the proper management response to it. Random variation in demand driven by clinical need is unavoidable, and tools appropriate for randomly arriving demand, such as queuing models, can

be employed to determine capacity needs. As stated in Chapter 4, artificial variability needs to be eliminated in order to maximize efficiency. A key question in patient flow analysis, then, is whether any variability found is random. In health care, the timing of many nonurgent services, such as elective surgeries and admissions, routine clinic visits, and many outpatient radiology procedures is determined in advance and scheduled by providers; variability in their timing is therefore not random but artificial. Therefore, it is essential to determine the contribution of scheduled versus unscheduled demand to total variability in the system.

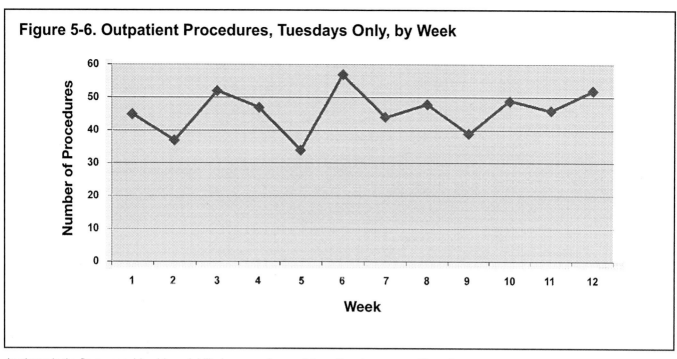

Figure 5-6. Outpatient Procedures, Tuesdays Only, by Week

As shown in the figure, considerable variability in case volume exists on Tuesdays across 12 weeks.

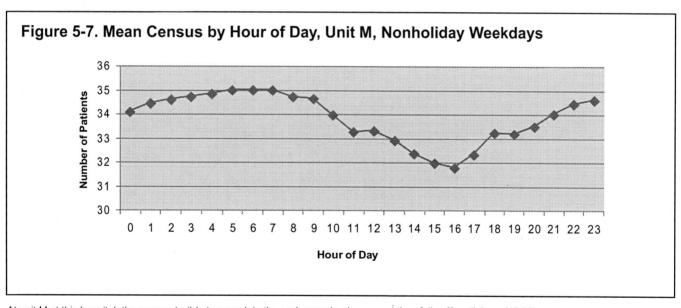

Figure 5-7. Mean Census by Hour of Day, Unit M, Nonholiday Weekdays

At unit M at this hospital, the census builds to a peak in the early morning hours and then falls off until 4 P.M. (16:00).

Unfortunately, health care information systems do not always capture data on scheduled versus unscheduled demand, although sometimes this variable can be constructed from other existing data. For example, admissions originating in the ED are generally (if not always) unscheduled, while patients admitted for elective surgeries are safely considered scheduled demand. Similarly, clinics may schedule some routine visits weeks or even months in advance, while they also experience patients requiring same-day visits for their acute needs. Although such visits may be in one sense "scheduled," in that a specific time for their visit is sug-

gested when they call, such demand is best understood as random because the ability to delay care to a more convenient (to the provider) or operationally efficient time is very limited.

Figure 5-13 (*see* page 84) suggests the type of analysis that is needed. Although in this example the relationship between elective and total demand is visually clear, it is often useful to determine the correlation coefficient (r) between total demand and its components to better understand the relationship. This is easily done using basic statistical software or even in an Excel spreadsheet,

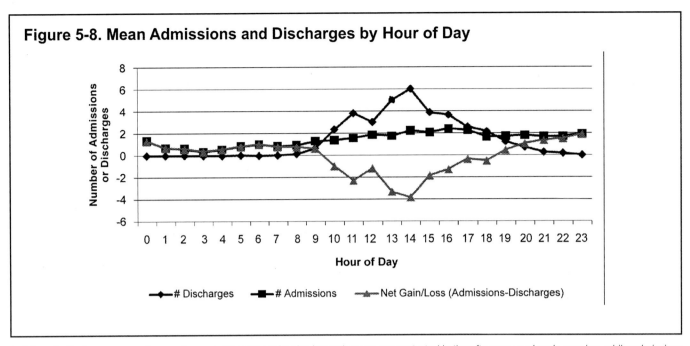

Figure 5-8. Mean Admissions and Discharges by Hour of Day

In this unit, discharges are not occurring smoothly across the day but rather are concentrated in the afternoon and early evening, while admissions are occurring around the clock (0 = midnight, 12 = noon).

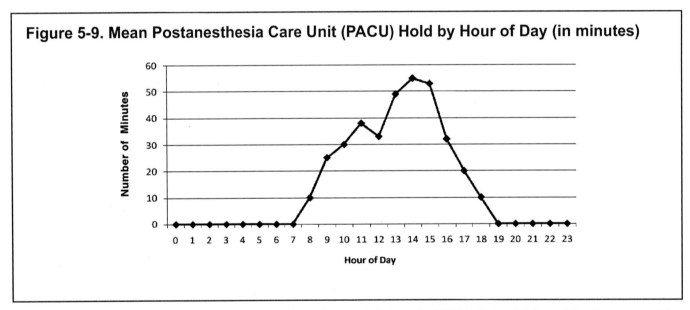

Figure 5-9. Mean Postanesthesia Care Unit (PACU) Hold by Hour of Day (in minutes)

This figure, which shows the mean wait for an inpatient bed by patients ready to leave the PACU, indicates that the wait time increases and then decreases, as beds in the nursing units are freed up and the elective surgery schedule is completed (0 = midnight, 12 = noon).

using the CORREL function, although Excel does not provide a calculation of statistical significance.

Similar types of analyses are useful for distinguishing the contribution of elective admissions to variability in total admissions or census, either by date or DOW. The admissions across the seven days of the week, as shown in Figure 5-14 (page 85), indicate a drop-off in new patients on weekends, as elective admissions or procedures diminish or disappear. However, where patients tend to have LOS of several days in length, census will not drop off as

dramatically as do admissions on the weekends (*see* Figure 5-15, page 85).

Sometimes there may be some doubt about whether variability in a given demand stream is truly random or whether there might be some artificial component. It is possible to test the pattern statistically to determine whether it deviates substantially from a random pattern of arrivals, which would fit a Poisson distribution. Some statistical software packages offer this capability, but it is also possible to do this calculation using Excel. Detailed instructions

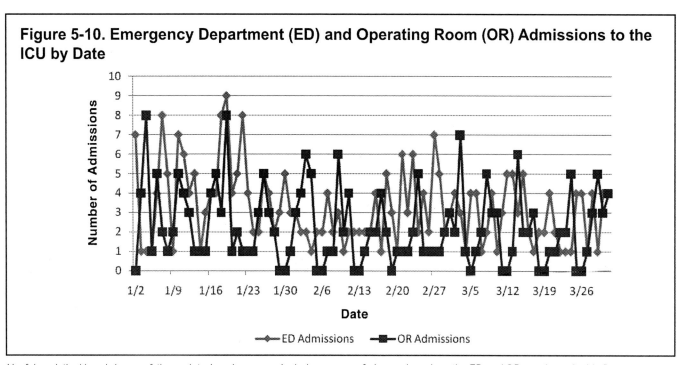

Figure 5-10. Emergency Department (ED) and Operating Room (OR) Admissions to the ICU by Date

Useful analytical breakdowns of time-related analyses may include sources of demand, such as the ED and OR, as shown in this figure.

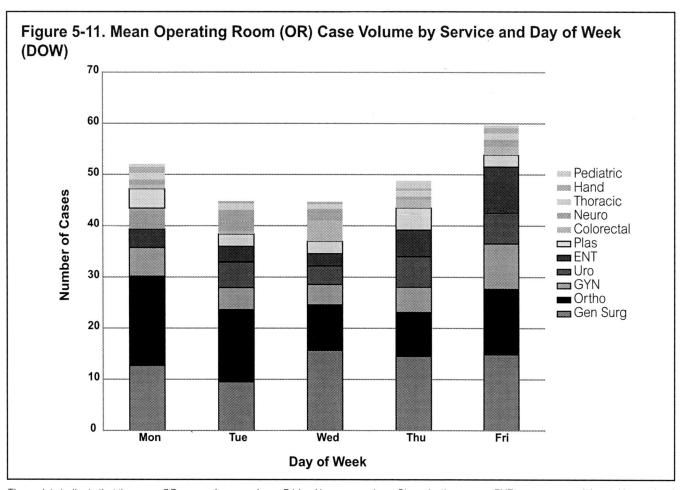

Figure 5-11. Mean Operating Room (OR) Case Volume by Service and Day of Week (DOW)

These data indicate that the mean OR case volume peaks on Friday. Neuro, neurology; Plas, plastic surgery; ENT, ears, nose, and throat; Uro, urology; GYN, gynecology; Ortho, orthopedic surgery; Gen Surg, general surgery. (The breakdown by service on the bars would be distinguished in color.)

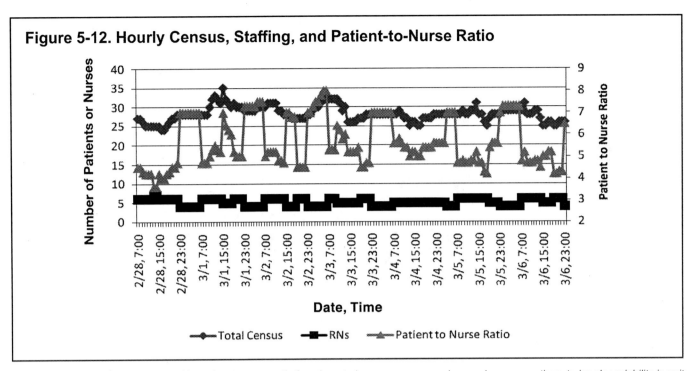

Figure 5-12. Hourly Census, Staffing, and Patient-to-Nurse Ratio

This figure portrays changes in a unit's patient-to-nurse ratio from hour to hour across seven days and compares them to hourly variability in unit census and staffing levels. RN, registered nurse.

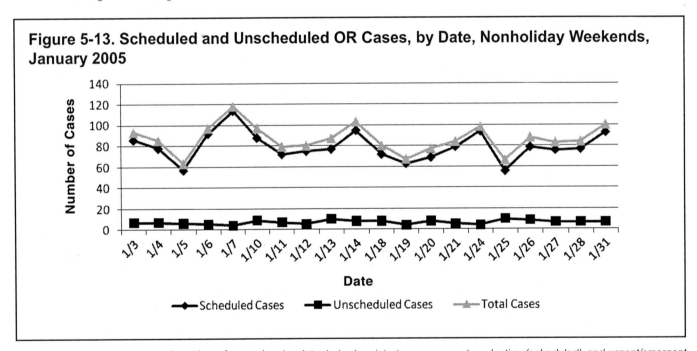

Figure 5-13. Scheduled and Unscheduled OR Cases, by Date, Nonholiday Weekends, January 2005

As shown in this figure, the total number of surgeries, by date, is broken into two components—elective (scheduled) and urgent/emergent (unscheduled)—for nonholiday weekdays in January 2005.

are provided in Sidebar 5-1 (*see* pages 86–87). Remember that what should be expected is that the *true demand* (Figure 5-1) for an unscheduled service would be random. If the available data are missing some patients who were diverted, and so on, and include others who do not belong, the test may provide spurious results.

Services Provided

To fully understand patient flow patterns, we need to explore not only timing patterns but other issues concerning the services provided to patients, including the following:

■ What care is needed? What care is actually provided?
■ How long does it take?

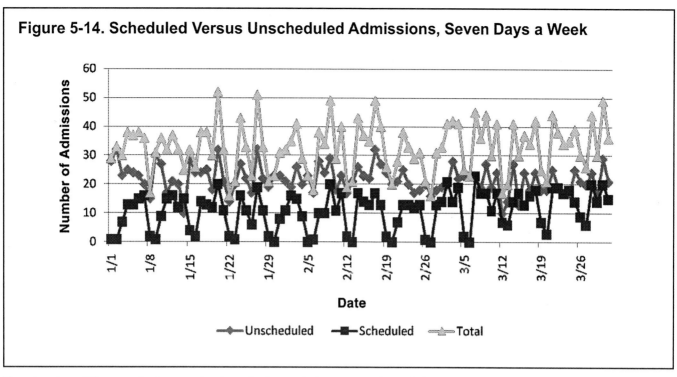

There is a drop-off in new patients on weekends as elective admissions or procedures diminish or disappear.

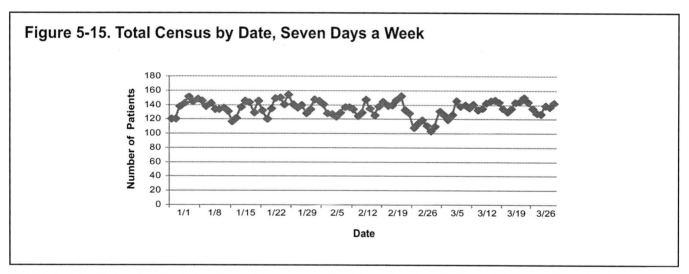

When patients tend to have lengths of stay of several days, census will not drop off as dramatically as admissions on the weekends.

■ Does the patient have to wait? If so, why?

The distinction between care that the patient *needs* and care that is *delivered* was raised earlier, in the discussion of typically available data on demand for specific patient care services. Clear admissions criteria or similar standards for other types of services (for example, for determining which laboratory test or imaging procedure is suitable for which patients) enable measurement of the gap between preferred care and actual care delivered—in general or for specific populations or over time. For example, differences in the proportions of patients who are admitted to their preferred

units, as shown in Figure 5-16 (page 87) may indicate possible capacity problems—but could also indicate greater or lesser variability in scheduling patterns that affect the hospital's ability to provide an appropriate bed. Drilling down a little more, exploring DOW patterns for specific services or for specific demand streams of patients can help to diagnose the cause of patient "misplacements." Figure 5-17 (page 88), for example, indicates that general surgeons at the hospital have much greater success sending their patients to the preferred unit on some weekdays than on others. Further exploration would be needed to assess the cause—for example, a tendency to have peak census on the unit late in the

Sidebar 5-1. Test for Randomness of Arrivals

Problem

We frequently want to know if the variability in an arrival pattern is due to fluctuations in a random process of arrivals, which would follow a Poisson distribution,[1] or whether it is due to artificial sources of variability. This question is important because the approach to dealing with the observed variability is different when the source is random than when it is artificial. An observed pattern of arrivals can be tested mathematically to determine whether it is statistically likely to be random.

Statistical Testing

One characteristic of a Poisson distribution is that the mean equals the variance. Thus, the first test we would want to do is a comparison of the observed mean and variance of our data. However, these will rarely be exactly equal, especially given the relatively small samples we work with. Therefore, we need another test for the randomness of the pattern of arrivals in our data.

The appropriate test to use is the chi-square test.[2] This test measures the "goodness of fit" between an observed pattern of arrivals and the expected pattern, given a Poisson process. The frequency at which each number of arrivals occurs over the period of observation (e.g., on how many days do 25 patients arrive? 26 patients? 27 patients? etc.) is compared with the frequency that would be expected with a Poisson process with:

- The same *mean* number of arrivals
- The same number of observations

The chi-square test indicates the probability that the differences between the observed and expected frequencies are great enough that they are probably not due to chance. A higher value of the chi-square statistic indicates that the null hypothesis (i.e., that the observed frequencies are not significantly different from expected frequencies) is disproved. Excel returns the *p* value, so that smaller values of the *p* value indicate statistical significance, depending on the cutoff selected.

One major limitation for our purposes is that the chi-square test is appropriate when the expected values of each frequency are at least 2 and most are 5 or more. Because we deal with relatively small numbers of observations, this can be a problem. However, in many cases we could combine adjacent cells to reach the cell sizes needed to use this test.

How to Perform the Test

1. Calculate the mean number of arrivals in the sample data. This will be used as the mean of a Poisson distribution for comparison purposes.

2. Note the number of observations (i.e., how many dates are included in the sample data?).

3. On an Excel worksheet, create a list of numbers ranging from 0 to the maximum value seen in the data. These numbers will be your "bins." Label the last value with a plus sign to indicate that it covers the last value to infinity

4. Calculate the *frequencies* at which each count of arrivals occurs—i.e., how many days fall into each bin—by one of the following methods:

   a. Histogram function:

      i. In the Tools menu, select Data Analysis. Then select histogram. Indicate:

         1. The range of data that needs to be analyzed
         2. The location of your list of bins
         3. Where you want the output to go

      ii. The output will replicate the list of bins and indicate the frequency at which each is found in the data. These are the OBSERVED frequencies.

   b. PivotTable:

      i. Use the date in the data field

      ii. Use the observed # of arrivals in the row field

      iii. Set the table to count the number of times each specific # of arrivals occurs. These are the OBSERVED frequencies.

5. Calculate the *probability* of each frequency in the list of bins with a Poisson process, given a certain mean. This is done using the Poisson function in Excel:

   a. Copy the list of bins to a new area of the worksheet.

   b. Select the cell to the right of the first value in the column of bins. Choose the Poisson function. Indicate:

      i. X = the particular bin for which we are calculating the probability. Indicate by selecting the cell to the left.

      ii. Mean = the sample mean

      iii. Type *false* so that the function returns the specific probability for each bin, not a cumulative probability.

      iv. Press Enter.

   c. Copy this cell downward so that probabilities are calculated for each bin. However, the value for the last cell (for the bin including infinity) should equal 1 minus the sum of all the other probabilities.

6. Calculate the EXPECTED frequencies, given the number of observations we have, using the probabilities just calculated for each bin:

   a. In the cell to the right of the calculated probability for the first bin, multiply the cell containing the probability value for that bin by the number of observations.

b. Copy this cell downward to calculate the expected values for all the bins.

7. Assemble the results and check the accuracy of the calculations:

a. Create a table with three columns:

i. The bins

ii. The observed values. Use 0 for each bin in which there are no observations in the sample.

iii. The expected values

b. Confirm that the sum of the expected values equals the sum of the observed values.

8. Evaluate cell size for the EXPECTED values; each should be ≥2, and most should be ≥ 5. Revise the table as necessary.

a. Combine adjacent cells to reach the threshold. This will most likely be necessary at both ends of the distribution, and possibly elsewhere as well.

b. Remember to combine the observed values to match the combined expected values and to label appropriately.

9. Run a chi-square test on the revised data table, using the CHITEST function in Excel. Indicate:

a. The range of the observed frequencies

b. The range of the expected frequencies

10. Interpret the output:

a. Excel provides the probability that the observed pattern could have been produced by chance using a Poisson process; smaller values thus indicate statistical significance.

Use $p = .05$ as the cutoff.

References

1. Gross D., et al.: *Fundamentals of Queueing Theory,* 4th ed. Hoboken, NJ: Wiley, 2008.

2. Neter J., Wasserman W., Whitmore G.A.: *Applied Statistics.* Boston: Allyn & Bacon Inc., 1978.

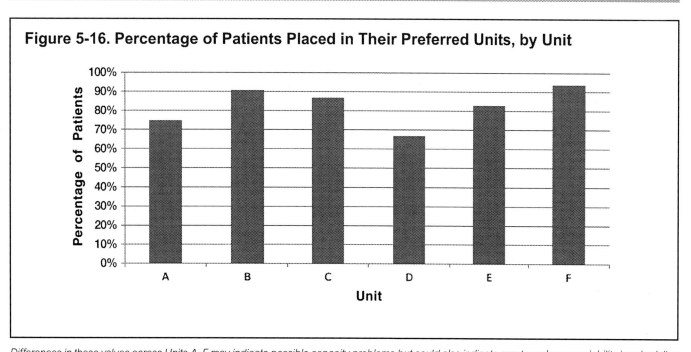

Figure 5-16. Percentage of Patients Placed in Their Preferred Units, by Unit

Differences in these values across Units A–F may indicate possible capacity problems but could also indicate greater or lesser variability in scheduling patterns that affect the hospital's ability to provide an appropriate bed.

week because of the accumulation of elective admissions, or, alternatively, overflows onto the given unit of patients who cannot be accommodated on their own preferred units.

Many of the analyses described so far have focused on counts of admissions, surgeries, tests, and so on. However, the needs of individual patients are not identical, and some patients absorb more resources than others, whether we are focusing on inpatient LOS,

time in the OR or PACU, clinic appointment length, or other variables. So merely counting patients is not enough. For management of patient flow, a key variable is the length of time it takes to treat a patient—that is, "service time." Furthermore, we need to know how good we are at predicting service time in advance.

With regard to admissions, it is informative to look at the overall distribution of LOS, whether in the hospital as a whole or for particular units (*see* Figure 5-18, page 89). Often, at least some of the variation in LOS is predictable, in that certain types of patients will have different mean LOS, whether they are grouped by diagnosis-related group procedure type, admission type (elective versus emergency), age, or other relevant variable (*see* Table 5-1, page 89). It follows logically that patients with a long mean LOS will have an impact on the hospital that is out of proportion to their volume of admissions. Therefore, it is useful to look not only at the percentage of admissions (or procedures, and so on) that patients of various types constitute but also the percentage of total bed days that they consume. As illustrated in Figure 5-19 (*see* page 90), a small number of patients can sometimes absorb a surprisingly large fraction of total resources or vice versa.

Similar issues are relevant to analysis of patient flow in the OR or the clinic. Thus, although total surgical minutes per day are usually correlated with patient counts, the relationship is not necessarily perfect (*see* Figure 5-20, page 90). Low surgical volume on certain days may be related to a concentration of long cases on those days; total surgical minutes can be more or less variable than the volume of cases performed. In the clinic, concentration of certain visit types during certain sessions may mean that fewer patients are seen on some days than others, even if total session time, cancellation rate, and so on are the same. In addition to patient or treatment type, variations in service length can also be linked to who is providing the service. Some physicians may simply spend more time with their patients during a visit or to

perform a procedure than do others, although it is important to control for case mix in any such analysis.

One issue with the quality of service time data is that these data may include some time that the patient spends waiting for the next step in care, even if treatment at the step being measured is complete. One common example is ED LOS. For admitted patients, the ED LOS is often extended because no inpatient bed is immediately available when the decision to admit is made. Other, perhaps less obvious, examples include the wait between the time a patient is ready to move out of the ICU to a floor unit and the time a bed becomes available for that patient, or the delay between the time the patient is ready to leave a unit and the time someone comes to transport him or her home. Although boarding time is certainly of interest for those concerned with hospital performance, it should be excluded from calculation of service time if the purpose is to determine and allocate capacity across the system to improve flow because it tends to exaggerate the resources needed.

Waits and Delays

We often need to address not only when the patient presents for or requests care but also when the treatment or care actually occurs. The difference between these two points in time represents the wait for service, which is of particular interest when the patient need is urgent. As indicated earlier, identification and measurement of patient waits for service throughout the system

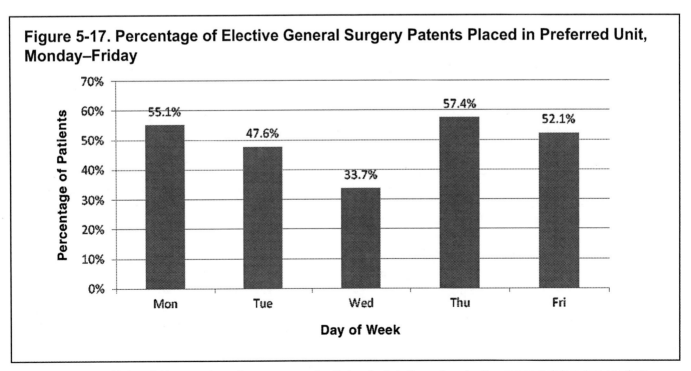

Figure 5-17. Percentage of Elective General Surgery Patents Placed in Preferred Unit, Monday–Friday

General surgeons at this hospital have much greater success sending their patients to the preferred unit on some weekdays than on others.

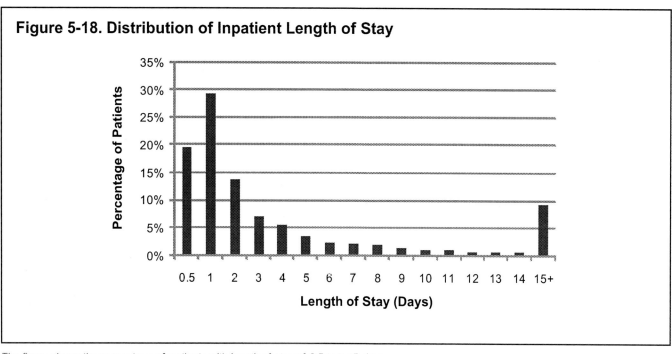

Figure 5-18. Distribution of Inpatient Length of Stay

The figure shows the percentage of patients with length of stay of 0.5 to ≥ 15 days.

Table 5-1. Diagnosis-Related Group (DRG), Admissions, and Length of Stay*

DRG	DRG Description	No. of Admissions	% Admissions	Mean LOS
127	Heart Failure & Shock	956	2.53%	5.08
544	Major Joint Replacement or Reattachment of Lower Extremity	897	2.37%	3.68
143	Chest Pain	778	2.06%	1.64
430	Psychoses	666	1.76%	10.35
557	Percutaneous Cardiovascular Procedure with Drug-Eluting Stent with Major Cardiovascular Diagnosis	624	1.65%	3.37
182	Esophagitis, Gastroenteritis & Miscellaneous Digestive Disorders Age > 17 with Complications & Comorbidities	565	1.49%	4.21
316	Renal Failure	532	1.41%	5.92
558	Percutaneous Cardiovascular Procedure with Drug-Eluting Stent Without Major Cardiovascular Diagnosis	529	1.40%	1.63
089	Simple Pneumonia & Pleurisy Age > 17 with Complications & Comorbidities	519	1.37%	4.62
088	Chronic Obstructive Pulmonary Disease	448	1.18%	4.56

*Data for one hospital for one year. LOS, length of stay.

can be extremely useful in determining where the blockages to smooth patient flow are occurring. Better collection of waiting or boarding times across the system would assist tremendously in diagnosis of patient flow problems, but few hospitals do this consistently. However, where data do exist or can be collected, they should be analyzed.

Chronic overcrowding in many EDs has provided a strong incentive for collecting data on the timing of various steps in the care process and on patient waits—for example, when the patient is placed in a treatment room, seen by a physician, or placed in an inpatient bed. Data on waits and delays also are often captured in the OR and PACU. In fact, delays in surgery start times are a

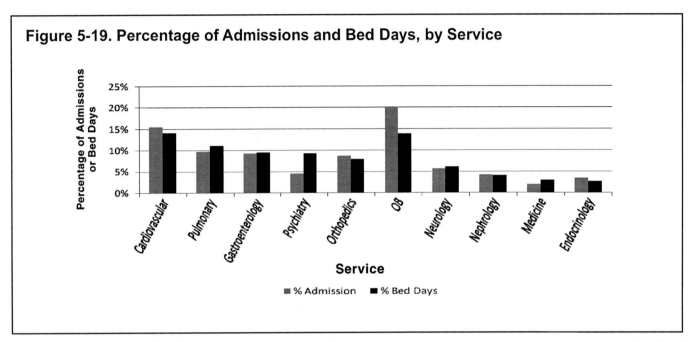

Figure 5-19. Percentage of Admissions and Bed Days, by Service

As shown in the figure, a small number of patients, as indicated by % admission), can sometimes consume a surprisingly large fraction of total resources (% Bed Days). OB, obstetrics.

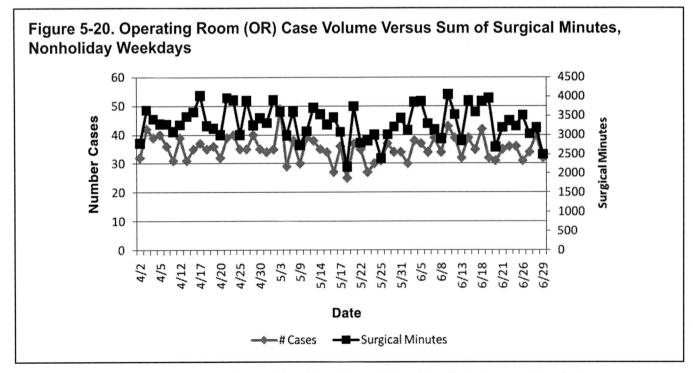

Figure 5-20. Operating Room (OR) Case Volume Versus Sum of Surgical Minutes, Nonholiday Weekdays

Although total surgical minutes per day are usually correlated with patient counts, the relationship is not necessarily perfect.

frequent complaint of unhappy surgeons but are also a quality of care issue, at least for some patients—those who need emergency or urgent procedures. If the hospital has established standards for acceptable maximum waits (that is, the patient would not be expected to be harmed if the procedure is performed within the standard) for procedures of various kinds, measuring the mean and median wait between the time the surgeon requests an OR and the time an OR is made available to him or her, as well as the number of failures to meet the standard, is a very good measure of timely access to care for that population (*see* Table 5-2, below).

It is also useful to perform an analysis to examine when during the day surgeries for urgent cases are usually performed (*see* Figure 5-21, below). If few such surgeries are performed during prime

time, and they instead cluster into overtime, then this is a sign that adequate resources to manage these patients during the day are not in place and that their timely flow through the system is blocked.

Determining why delays occur will help to identify solutions to patient flow blockages; collecting data on reasons for delays, and not merely their occurrence, can be very helpful. Sometimes delays reflect poor "discipline," as when patients or providers do not arrive on time for appointments or procedures. Sometimes they reflect poor planning or scheduling practices—for example, when surgeons systematically underestimate predicted case length in order to squeeze one more case into their block time schedule (*see* Figure 5-22, page 92), or when clinic staff double-book the schedule to accommodate additional patient visits. Scheduling

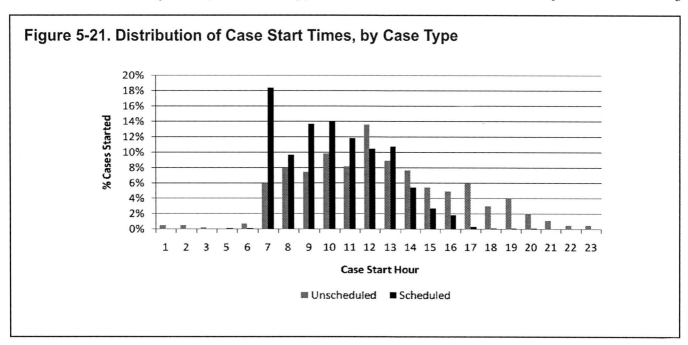

Figure 5-21. Distribution of Case Start Times, by Case Type

The data in this figure indicate that while surgery is performed for most scheduled cases earlier in the day, many unscheduled cases begin after the usual operating room workday ends.

Table 5-2. Waiting Time for Surgery*

Maximum Wait Standard	Median Wait (hr:min)	Mean Wait (hr:min)	Percent Failures
1 hour	0:23	0:29	7%
4 hours	2:02	2:47	9%
12 hours	6:41	8:07	10%
24 hours	14:54	17:23	6%

*Hr, hour; min, minutes.

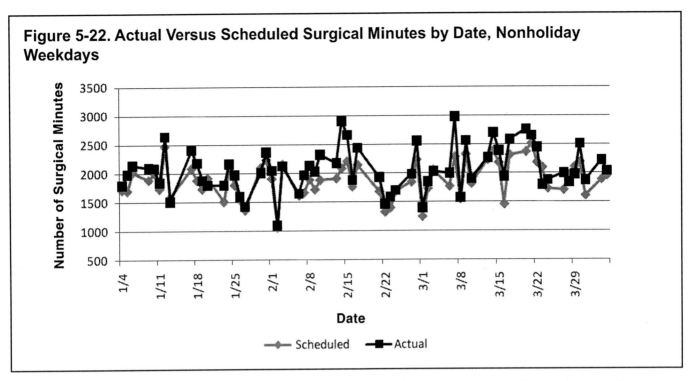

Figure 5-22. Actual Versus Scheduled Surgical Minutes by Date, Nonholiday Weekdays

In this OR, actual surgical minutes usually exceed scheduled surgical minutes, indicating a bias toward underestimation of case length when cases are scheduled.

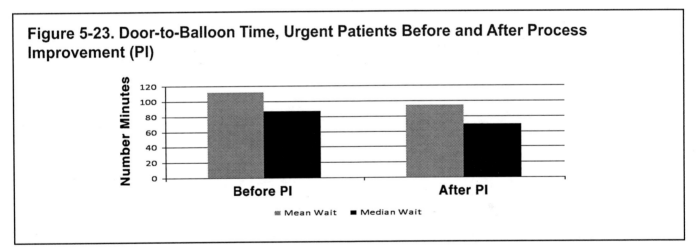

Figure 5-23. Door-to-Balloon Time, Urgent Patients Before and After Process Improvement (PI)

Data were collected for a comparison of waits by acutely ill patients for access to the cardiac catheterization laboratory—before and after an intervention to improve the timeliness of care.

systems often permit selection of a limited set of scheduled procedure or visit durations, such as in 15-minute intervals, which will not necessarily be the best fit to actual experience. In addition, sometimes delays are due to major bottlenecks in flows through the system, such as when the ED slows down because it is full of admitted patients for whom no available inpatient beds exist, thus reducing its effective capacity to treat new patients.

Of course, from a quality of care point of view, the significance of a given wait depends on whether it increases the risk to the patient. Although some waits, such as for interunit transfers to

equal or lower levels of care, or for discharge, may be of concern primarily for efficiency reasons (although care of other patients needing beds may be delayed or blocked because of the resulting increased LOS), where the clinical need is urgent, as for emergency surgery or for many ED admissions, longer waits equal lower quality of care. Such waits are important to track and measure, and where the hospital has set standards, success in meeting them should be tracked, as shown in Figure 5-23 (above).

When the service (for example, radiology examination) is scheduled in advance, it is useful to compare the actual start times with

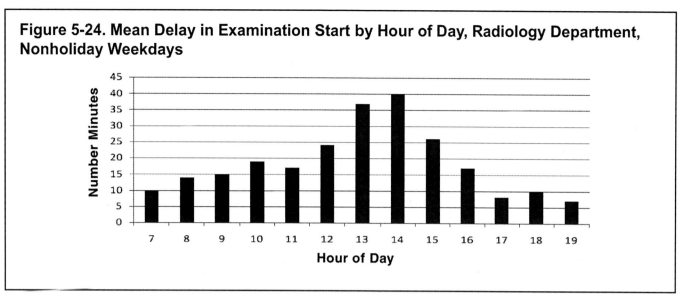

Figure 5-24. Mean Delay in Examination Start by Hour of Day, Radiology Department, Nonholiday Weekdays

As the data in the figure show, mean waits tend to increase across the hours of the day until midafternoon, after which they decrease.

scheduled start times. Comparing the mean waits across hour of the day might show that delays and waits tend to grow as the day goes on because late-starting visits, examinations, or procedures tend to end late as well, and the effect can be cumulative until the point at which volume drops off (*see* Figure 5-24, above).

Sometimes delays occur because of systemic flow problems, such as when the PACU fills with patients and is unable to discharge them because discharges have not yet occurred on the floors, so that the OR backs up as well. These are the sorts of issues that analysis of well-specified delay codes can illuminate.

Conclusion

Collection and analysis of accurate data are necessary for the assessment of the current state of patient flow in a hospital and for the design of strategies to manage patient flow more effectively. Awareness of potential quality problems with existing data sets will help to avoid misinterpretation of analyses. Yet the data needed to perform many informative analyses are readily available through most health care information systems. For the future, capture of additional data on waits and delays (possibly with the assistance of radio frequency identification device technology), the urgency of patients' clinical needs, and the appropriateness of the care provided will permit even deeper insight into the measurement and analysis of patient flow.

Reference

1.   Neter J., Wasserman W., Whitman G.A.: *Applied Statistics.* Boston: Allyn & Bacon Inc., 1978.

Section II. Case Studies

Chapter 6

Cincinnati Children's Hospital Medical Center: Redesigning Perioperative Flow Using Operations Management Tools to Improve Access and Safety

Frederick C. Ryckman, M.D.; Elena Adler, M.D.; Amy M. Anneken, M.S.; Cindi A. Bedinghaus, R.N., M.S.N.; Peter J. Clayton, M.P.A.; Kathryn R. Hays, M.S.N., R.N.; Brenda Lee; Jacquelyn W. Morillo-Delerme, M.D.; Pamela J. Schoettker, M.S.; Paul A. Yelton; Uma R. Kotagal, M.B.B.S., M.Sc.

Waits, delays, and cancellations have become so common in health care that both patients and providers assume that waiting is an inevitable part of the process.[1] Nevertheless, such symptoms of disrupted patient flow through the health care system result in enormous frustration to patients, families, and staff. Disrupted patient flow has a negative effect on patient satisfaction, staff retention, referrals, and reimbursement, and, most importantly, it has a direct impact on patient safety. Patient congestion has been associated with treatment delays, medical errors, and unsafe practices that can lead to adverse events and poorer outcomes.[2–5] In addition, patients being placed on the wrong care unit or unable to transfer to the appropriate unit are precursor events to safety failures.

Cincinnati Children's Hospital Medical Center

Cincinnati Children's Hospital Medical Center, the only pediatric hospital in the greater Cincinnati area, serves as a primary referral center for an eight-county area in southwestern Ohio, northern Kentucky, and southeastern Indiana. In fiscal year 2008 (July 2007–June 2008), Cincinnati Children's had 27,392 admissions and 93,456 emergency department (ED) visits and performed 6,323 inpatient surgical procedures and 22,845 outpatient surgical procedures during 43,325 surgical hours in 20 rooms. The 25-bed pediatric intensive care unit (ICU) had an average daily census of 17 children in 2006, 20 in 2007, and 21 in 2008.

Identifying the Problem

Like other health care organizations, Cincinnati Children's has had problems with delays in care and poor patient flow through the system. As the hospital has grown and expanded, the number of referrals from across the United States and the world has increased, as has the complexity of the care required. Emergency surgeries were considered unpredictable and were done at the end of the day or forced into slots between scheduled cases. The result was a long list of add-on patients at the conclusion of the regular day and long waiting times for children with urgent needs. Complex cases were often done in the evening or at night, when resources were limited. The competition for available beds in the pediatric ICU sometimes resulted in patients being held in the ED or postanesthesia care unit, causing those locations to back up and causing elective surgeries to be delayed or cancelled. Patients sometimes were placed in beds that were not optimal for their condition. Wide swings in census were difficult to staff, resulting in long hours, fatigue, and reduced morale. Clinicians and families were left frustrated.

Cincinnati Children's has maintained a significant focus on transforming the care delivery system since the late 1990s.[6] In 2001, a new strategic plan aimed at dramatically improving the outcomes, value, and cost of care for children was launched. This plan committed the organization to sustaining breakthrough improvements in clinical outcomes, reducing medical errors, delivering cost-effective care, improving care coordination, and enhancing access to care and timeliness of services delivered. *Improving patient flow* was one of the six original strategic priorities established at a 2002 retreat attended by 100 faculty and organizational leaders.

Preliminary attempts to improve flow, such as increasing the staff in the ED to meet the expected increase in demand during bronchiolitis season, were made at the level of microsystems, the small work units that deliver the care that the patient experiences.[7] However, flow is a series of coordinated, interdependent systems, not the result of isolated independent systems. To truly change the way patients flowed through the care system, Cincinnati Children's chose to look outside health care to operations research methodologies widely used in many other industries, such as banking, insurance, manufacturing, transportation, military, and telecommunications.

The hospital's president and chief executive officer, James Anderson, along with the senior vice president for quality and transformation [U.R.K.], served as the project champions of the efforts to improve perioperative flow. In 2006, two of the authors [F.C.R., U.R.K.] met Eugene Litvak, Ph.D. (Program for Management of Variability in Health Care Delivery, Boston University Health Policy Institute, Boston), who, with his colleagues, has studied the effect of variability in patient flow on hospital operations and has described two types of variation in the demand for health care services.[8] There is random—sometimes called natural—variation in the types of diseases or injuries patients present with, their severity of illness, and their arrival patterns. Random variation is beyond the control of the health care system and so cannot be eliminated, but it can be optimally

managed. Nonrandom, or artificial, variation is related to the design and management of the way care is delivered or to the behavior of the primary health care providers. It is, thus, potentially controllable. When possible, nonrandom variability should be eliminated.[1] Research has shown that emergency presentations to the operating room (OR) follow a random demand pattern, while the day-to-day variation in elective surgical cases and scheduled requests for an ICU bed are artificial and controllable.[8,9] In addition, the effect of nonrandom, artificial variation on flow far exceeds the effect of natural variation.[8–10] Thus, patient flow can be improved by smoothing the surgical schedule.[1]

In the months preceding the start of this initiative, informal discussions among authors [F.C.R., U.R.K., P.J.C.] and leaders from the departments of surgery and anesthesia confirmed agreement that there were serious problems with patient flow in the OR. However, there was no consensus on the root of the problem. Without data to support opinions, delayed or postponed surgical cases were blamed on slow cleaning of rooms or late patients or surgeons. Because of the multilevel failure points, individual improvements, such as shifting cases or reorganizing the case schedule, that would transform the care in the perioperative area were common, but their lack of interdependent linkage meant that real improvement did not occur.

A New Start

To better serve patients, improve patient safety, and increase the efficiency and reliability of the care delivered,[11] in January 2007 Cincinnati Children's implemented a series of interventions to match demand and capacity to optimize timely, safe, and efficient care as patients flow through and between the Cincinnati Children's ED, perioperative services, or inpatient units, including the pediatric ICU and areas for diagnostic and therapeutic interventions. The specific goals of the interventions were to (1) identify and separate the urgent/emergent case flow from the elective surgical cases and to improve access and throughput and (2) smooth the inflow of elective admissions to the pediatric ICU to make bed occupancy more predictable. A prominent pediatric surgeon [F.C.R.], trained in improvement science, agreed to lead the flow initiative. He was supported by a small steering team, which included authors [E.A., A.M.A., C.A.B., P.J.C., K.R.H., B.L., J.W.M.-D., P.A.Y., U.R.K.] and James Anderson.

Measuring Patient Flow

The first step was to collect baseline data on the current flow through the OR and pediatric ICU. The importance of correct and precise data was recognized early in the project because the

Chapter 6: *Cincinnati Children's Hospital Medical Center: Redesigning Perioperative Flow Using Operations Management Tools to Improve Access and Safety*

99

flow models were to be constructed on the basis of the case data analysis. Because much of the needed information was not automated, data had to be collected by hand to establish the project. When initial attempts to collect data by individuals without health care training proved to be unreliable, Cincinnati Children's began using in-house employees with previous experience in process improvement. Retrospective data had to be confirmed and new service data validated. This process was time-consuming, and its duration and intensity strained the improvement fabric of the perioperative area.

Outcomes measures were related to delay in the system and included the following:
■ Volume of cases
■ OR utilization (the percentage of available elective surgical time that rooms were used)
■ Timeliness of add-on case (cases that required access to the OR within 24 hours and were not scheduled in advance) access to the OR (percentage of cases started within established goal time frames, measured from the time a case was requested until the time the case began)
■ Percentage of days that the OR went over scheduled time
■ Daily mean surgical elective cases in pediatric ICU beds
■ Daily mean surgical elective cases in cardiac ICU beds (considered diversions)
Clinicians were also surveyed about their experiences with add-on ORs.

Measures are presented in monthly reports and annotated control charts that are provided to the multidisciplinary perioperative clinical system improvement team (*right*), and organizational leadership and are also posted on the hospital's patient safety intranet site.

To improve electronic data collection and direct improvement efforts, Cincinnati Children's retooled the OR scheduling system to ask important flow-related questions, increasing the amount of work required to schedule a case. The additional information added to the scheduling system included prophylactic antibiotic management, case grouping for urgent/emergent add-on cases, ICU bed need and predicted ICU stay, and floor bed need and estimated stay. This information was obtained from individual physician offices and clinics and sent to the same-day surgery center as faxed orders.

In September 2002, Cincinnati Children's moved to a new building, at which point it implemented a system to integrate clinical information that included computerized clinical order entry, clinical documentation, an electronic medication administration record, a data storage repository, and advanced clinical decision support. The medical center is now implementing a new core clinical and financial information system developed by a commercial vendor. Flow measures are being integrated into the information system, and some of them are expected to "go live" in January 2010.

Implementation of Strategies
Planning. The multidisciplinary perioperative clinical system improvement team, formed in January 2005, was composed of key frontline staff from the departments of surgery, anesthesia, perioperative administration, and patient services. A quality improvement consultant and a data analyst from the division of health policy and clinical effectiveness provided support in the application of quality improvement science, data collection, and data analysis. The hospital's chief executive officer served as the team champion and ensured that the team received the help it needed to align the work with organizational priorities, overcome organizational barriers, identify resources, foster energy for change, and share results of activities.

To help build the will for changes to be made, experts from the Program for Management of Variability in Health Care Delivery came to Cincinnati Children's for a day of open sessions with senior leaders and all the surgeons. They made presentations at large- and small-group gatherings and one-on-one meetings. A major concern of the surgeons was that changes would be made to schedules that would result in a loss of patients and revenue; block times (designated times in specific ORs that are assigned or held for surgeons or surgical services for their exclusive use) would be changed, conflicting with established clinical office times; or conflicts would be created with preestablished academic commitments. Access to adequate block time to accomplish elective cases was also a major concern. The surgeons were assured that their time in the OR would not be limited. The goal was clearly articulated to be an improvement in access and care via control of unnatural variation in scheduling and urgent/emergent cases. Model data analysis was supplied by Dr. Litvak and his colleagues, and a close partnership with the program continued throughout the project. Existing Cincinnati Children's system analysts and data managers tracked changes in outcome measures over time. Although Cincinnati Children's did not hire any new employees to complete the project, it did redirect some of the other work that these individuals were responsible for so that they had the time and resources to work on this project.

As reported previously, key driver diagrams were developed to provide a framework of the proposed aim, key factors necessary for improvement, and potential change strategies to improve flow in the pediatric ICU (*see* Figure 6-1, page 100).[12]

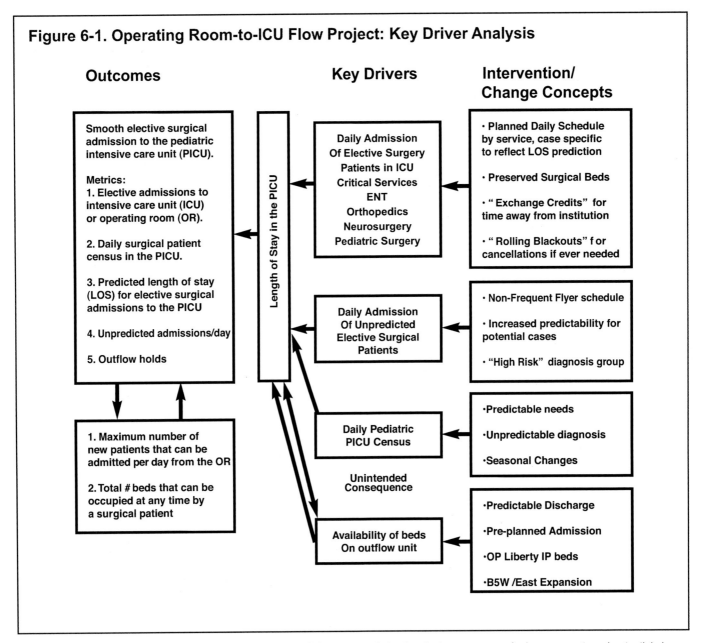

Figure 6-1. Operating Room-to-ICU Flow Project: Key Driver Analysis

Key driver diagrams were developed to provide a framework of the proposed aim, key factors necessary for improvement, and potential change strategies to improve flow in the pediatric intensive care unit. LOS, length of stay; ENT, ear, nose, throat; IP, inpatient. The intervention OP Liberty IP beds refers to a plan to add inpatient beds to a large outpatient facility.

Source: *Cincinnati Children's Hospital Medical Center. Used with permission.*

The interventions were steps to define the urgency of need on the basis of medical condition, risk, and rapidity of progression. Historical data were used to identify "streams" (risk groups). These were then assigned real volume and OR case times, which were used in prediction simulations to calculate how many ORs would be needed to accommodate the caseload. The system built and then incorporated the rules for stratifying the cases and running the caseload on a daily basis. The follow-up system was designed to measure the results against the time- and safety-based goals.

Dedication of ORs to Urgent/Emergent Cases. To allow more efficient booking of cases, better reliability of room utilization, and improved schedule predictability, the team decided to separate the stream of elective cases from the stream of emergency add-on cases by dedicating ORs each day for urgent/emergent cases. The first step was to achieve consensus on a definition of urgent and emergent cases. Toward that end, the team established time goals for safe patient access to the OR on the basis of five levels of clinical need:

Chapter 6: *Cincinnati Children's Hospital Medical Center: Redesigning Perioperative Flow Using Operations Management Tools to Improve Access and Safety*

101

- A: Acute life-and-death emergencies—into the OR in < 30 minutes
- B: Emergent but not immediately life-threatening—into the OR in < 2 hours
- C: Urgent—into the OR in < 4 hours
- D: Semiurgent—into the OR in < 8 hours
- E: Add-on case to elective schedule—into the OR in < 24 hours

Remaining unscheduled cases that needed access to the OR within 24 hours to 7 days were designated as work-in cases.

Surgical Chiefs' Classification of Cases as A–E.
Individual surgical chiefs for each surgical division were asked to classify all their cases according to the A to E categories. The improvement team then developed an urgency-based list of diagnoses and procedures, stratified according to the established time goals (*see* Table 6-1, below). This list was presented to providers

as a guideline only, noting that medical judgment was still required. At the beginning of the initiative, the list was updated almost monthly. More recently, new cases are added as they are defined. In addition, the list is updated at the request of services if they feel that their patient needs have changed.

Determination of Number of ORs for Urgent/Emergent Cases. To balance the elective and emergency workloads, discrete-event simulation models based on queuing theory were used to determine the optimal number of ORs to set aside for urgent/emergent cases. Separate models were created for weekdays (7:00 A.M. to midnight), weekends, and nights (midnight to 7:00 A.M.). The models considered the cases included (A to E), the number of rooms available, the average wait times, the probability that one or more rooms would be available, and the utilization rate. Cases where data were missing were classified as type

Table 6-1. Guidelines for Surgical Case Grouping by Diagnoses/Procedures*

Guideline only: medical judgment required

Acute Life and Death Emergencies

A **< 30 Minutes**

Airway emergency (upper airway obstruction)
Cardiac surgery postoperative bleeding with tamponade
Cardiorespiratory decompensation (severe)
Liver transplant postoperative emergency
Malrotation with volvulus
Massive bleeding
Mediastinal injury
MuffipleTrauma - unstable or O.R. resuscitation
Neurosurgical condition w/imminent herniation

Emergent, but not immediately life threatening

B **< 2 Hours**

Acute shunt malfunction
Acute spinal cord corn pression
Bladder rupture
Bowel perforation, traumatic
Cardiac congenital emergencies w/hemodynamic or pulmonary instabilities
Compartment syndrome
Donor harvest
ECMO cannulation
Ectopic pregnancy
Embolization for acute hemorrhage
Esophageal atresia with tracheoesophageal fistula
Gastroschisis/omphalocele
Heart; heart/lung, lung, liver and intestinal transplants
Incarcerated hernias
Intestinal obstruction with suspected vascular compromise
Intussusception-irreducible
Ischemic limb/cold extremity (compromised arterial flow)
Liver/ Multivisceral /SI Transplant (when organ available)
Liver transplant with suspected thrombosis
Newborn bowel obstruction
Open globe
Orbital abscess
Pacemaker insertion for complete heart block
Replant fingers
Replant hand or arm
Spontaneous abortion
Tonsil Bleed
Torsion of testis/ovary
Vascular compromises
Wound Dehiscence

Urgent **C** **< 4 Hours**

Abscess with sepsis
Airway (non-urgent diagnostic L&B, flex bronch, non-symptomatic foreign body)
Appendicitis-with sepsis/rapid progression
Biliary obstruction non-drainable
Cardiac ventricular assist device placement
Cerebral angiogram for intracranial hemorrhage
Chest tube placement in patient w/unstable vital signs, increased work of breathing and decreased oxygen saturation
Contaminated Wounds-MultipleTrauma
Diagnostic/therapeutic airway intervention
Hepatic angiogram w/suspected vascular thrombus
Hip Dislocation
Intestinal Obstruction-no suspected vascular compromise
Kidney transplant (ORGAN AVAILABLE)
Liver laparotomy
Massive soft tissue injury
Nephrostomy tube placement in patient w/sepsis
Obstructed kidney (stones) with sepsis
Older child with bowel obstruction
PICC placement where patient has no access but needs fluids/medications urgently
Progressive shunt malfunction
Traumatic dislocation-hip
Unstable neurosurgical condition

Semi-Urgent **D** **< 8 Hours**

Abscess drainage
Appendicitis-stable/elective
Caustic ingestion
Chest tube in patient w/stable vital signs
Chronic airway foreign bodies
Closure abdomen - liver transplant
Coarctation repair in newborn
Esophageal foreign body without airway symptoms
GJ tube/NJ tube placement with no other nutrition access
Hematuria with clot retention
I&D abscess without septicemia
Joint aspiration or bone biopsy prior to starting antibiotic therapy
Kidney transplant (ORGAN NOT YET AVAILABLE)
Liver/ Multivisceral /SI Transplant (ORGAN NOT YET AVAILABLE)
Nephrostomy tube placement
Obstructed kidney without sepsis
Open fracture grade III
Septic joint

Add-on case to elective schedule

E **< 24 Hours**

(Needs to be done that day, but does not require the manipulation of the elective schedule, i.e., pyloromyotomy)
Broviac
Closed reduction
Eyelid/ canalicular lacerations
Facial nerve decompression
Femoral neck fracture
Liver biopsy
Mastoidectomy
Open fracture grade I/II
Open reduction of fracture
PICC placement - has other IV access
Retinopathy of prematurity treatment
Unstable slipped capital femoral epiphysis

*L & B, laryngoscopy and bronchoscopy; OR, operating room; PICC, peripherally inserted central catheter; IV, intravenous; ECMO, extracorporeal membrane oxygenation; SI, small intestinal transplant; GJ, gastrojejunal; NJ, nasojejunal; I & D, incision and drainage.
Source: Cincinnati Children's Hospital Medical Center. Used with permission.

B in the models to be conservative regarding meeting the clinical need.

Selection of Models. Simulation models were selected by matching the appropriate timely access and safety goals, with the recognition that appropriate access for urgent/emergent cases dictated a lower utilization rate in those rooms.

The OR simulation models selected were as follows:

• *A to E Cases, Weekdays, 7:00 A.M. (07:00)–11:59 P.M. (23:59):* The best model recommended that two ORs be set aside for any A to E case (*see* Table 6-2, below). With this scenario, wait times were predicted to be 7 minutes for A cases, 8 minutes for B cases, 9 minutes for C and D cases, and 17 minutes for E cases. The probability that one or more rooms would be available was 83%, and the utilization rate would be 42% for each room. It was estimated that wait times for A cases would exceed the stated limit about 1 time in 112 weekdays (21.4 weeks).

• *A to E Cases, Weekends.* The best model recommended that two ORs be set aside for 7:00 A.M. (07:00)–6:59 P.M. (18:59) on Saturday and Sunday, with an additional trauma/A room on call if needed. With this scenario, average wait times were predicted to be 8 minutes for A and B cases, 9 minutes for C cases, and 12 minutes for D and E cases. The probability of one or more rooms being available would be 87%, and the utilization would be 36% for each room.

• *Weekday Nights.* The best model recommended that one room be set aside for A to D cases, midnight (24:00)–6:59 A.M. (06:59). With this scenario, average wait times were predicted to be 22 minutes for A cases, 24 minutes for B cases, 27 minutes for C cases, and 31 minutes for D cases. E cases were excluded during this time period. The probability that one or more rooms would be available would be 81%, and the utilization rate would be 19%. It was estimated that a room will not be immediately available for an A case once every six months.

• *Weekend Nights.* The best model recommended that one room be set aside for A to D cases, 7:00 P.M. (19:00)–6:59 A.M. (06:59). Average wait times were estimated to be 19 minutes for A cases, 20 minutes for B cases, 22 minutes for C cases, and 24 minutes for D cases. E cases were excluded during this time

Table 6-2. Models for Cases A–E, Weekdays, 7:00 A.M. (07:00)–11:59 P.M. (23:59)

#	Cases Included	# Rooms	Average Waiting Times (minutes)	Probability 1 Or More Rooms Will Be Available	Utilization Rate	Recommendations/Considerations
1	A, B, C, D, "missing" treated as B	1	A : 45 B + missing: 53 C: 72 D: 101	60%	40%	NOT RECOMMENDED 1. Mean wait for A cases would exceed stated limit
2	A, B, C, "missing" treated as B	1	A: 21 B + missing: 24 C: 30	76%	24%	NOT RECOMMENDED 1) Low utilization rate
3	A, B, C (No "missing")	1	A: 17 B: 19 C: 22	81%	19%	NOT RECOMMENDED 1) Low utilization rate 2) Ignores "missing" cases
4	A – E, divided; "missing" treated as D	2 rooms: 1 room for A - C, 1 room for D, E, & missing	A: 18 B: 19 C: 24 D + missing: 70 E: 162	A – C room: 80% D – E room: 43%	A – C room: 20% D – E room: 57%	NOT RECOMMENDED 1) Low utilization rate in A – C room 2) Some cases with missing urgency codes may be more urgent than D
5	A – E together; "missing" treated as B	2 rooms that would take any A – E case	A: 7 B + missing: 8 C + D: 9 E: 17	83%	42%, each room	**RECOMMENDED** 1) Very good waiting times (Wait for A cases would exceed stated limit about 1X/112 weekdays (21.4 weeks)) 2) Treats missing cases conservatively 3) Highest utilization rate 4) Not very sensitive to small increases in case duration or case volume

Source: Cincinnati Children's Hospital Medical Center. Used with permission.

Chapter 6: *Cincinnati Children's Hospital Medical Center: Redesigning Perioperative Flow Using Operations Management Tools to Improve Access and Safety*

103

period. With this scenario, the probability that one or more rooms would be available would be 84%, and the utilization rate would be 16%. It was estimated that a room will not be immediately available for an A case once every five years.

Determining Surgeon Availability. Surgeon availability was addressed by individual divisions using different methods. For divisions with frequent add-on cases and urgent needs, such as pediatric general surgery, orthopedics, and otolaryngology, a dedicated surgeon was identified each day or week. Although this surgeon had other responsibilities, his or her primary responsibility was to be available for urgent and emergent cases. Divisions with lesser needs or a small staff component used an on-call system. Although their availability was more limited, the ability to clear other high-frequency add-ons from the schedule in a timely fashion made it more likely that a room would be available when their needs arose.

Testing of Models for the Pediatric ICU. A new prediction pathway for patients in the pediatric ICU was tested on the basis of the surgeons' predicted need for ICU care and length of stay (LOS) obtained from the baseline data. The prediction pathway originally served as a "single-shot" prediction model. That is, on the day the procedure was scheduled, surgeons were asked to make a one-time prediction of how long the patient was expected to be in the ICU. Ongoing interventions include making it available at the bedside as a computer model that can be used to update the predictions daily as a patient's care evolves. It now also stores information on the preferred location for patients after they leave the ICU to assist in demand-capacity matching to the floor beds.

Revision of the Surgical Scheduling System. The surgical scheduling system was revised so that the OR and ICU bed were scheduled simultaneously for surgical cases requiring an ICU bed. In addition, a projected LOS in the pediatric ICU was established when the case was initially scheduled. Posted beds were continuously monitored, and the computerized scheduling system restricted case scheduling if the pediatric ICU elective case limit for that day had been reached.

Morning Huddle. A morning huddle—a daily 6 A.M. (06:00) meeting of the chief of staff, manager of patient services, and representatives from the OR, pediatric ICU, and anesthesia—is held to confirm the plan for that day and anticipate the needs for the next day. Over time, this strategy has broadened to include discharge prediction of outflow units, allowing better proactive demand-capacity matching for patients transferred from the pediatric ICU to patient floors and for opening beds for the predicted incoming surgical patients.

Matching Capacity to Demand. On the basis of the OR models, 85% of all OR time was allocated to physician-specific blocks, two add-on rooms were set aside each day for A–E cases, and one room was set aside for work-in cases needing access in less than seven days (*see* Figure 6-2, page 104). Correct classification was confirmed by the surgical scheduler when the case was scheduled.

When the add-on/work-in room allocations were set, they were integrated with preexisting call schedule requirements (for example, Level 1 trauma room availability, specialty call, allowing a set plan for staffing the entire OR at all hours). The preestablished, agreed-on, safety-directed waiting times for add-on cases clearly identified the need for calling in on-call additional resources to meet the rare, but occasional, increased need. This removed the emotional component from calling in colleagues at night and on weekends because the decision was based on the mathematics of the urgent/emergent add-on system, not individual choice.

Results

Smoothing OR Flow

As a result of the redesign, weekday waiting times were decreased by 28%, despite a 24% increase in case volume (*see* Figure 6-3, page 105, which shows wait time for A cases; "Timeliness of add-ons," as listed on page 99). On the weekends, waiting times decreased by 34%, despite a 37% increase in case volume. Overall, growth in case volume was sustained at approximately 7% per year for the next two years ("Volume of cases").

Overtime hours decreased by an estimated 57% between September 18, 2006, and the first week of January 2007 ("Percent of days that the OR went over scheduled time"). If OR operating costs are estimated at $250/room hour, then these savings are equivalent to $10,750/week, or $559,000 annually.

The true value of redesign for increased efficiency can best be appreciated by contrasting it to the costs of building new resources. Throughput, the total number of case hours during a routine OR day, increased 4.8% ("OR utilization"). This is nearly equivalent to the addition of one more OR, without any of the associated capital or operating costs.

Initial improvements in staffing were achieved as late overtime rooms were no longer necessary. Emergency case volume was accommodated during prime working hours, decreasing the need for complex surgical intervention after hours. Since the initiation of the changes in 2006, overtime hours as a percentage of total hours decreased by 19% during fiscal year 2008 and an additional 15% during fiscal year 2009.

Figure 6-2. Comparison of the Old and New Surgical Scheduling Models

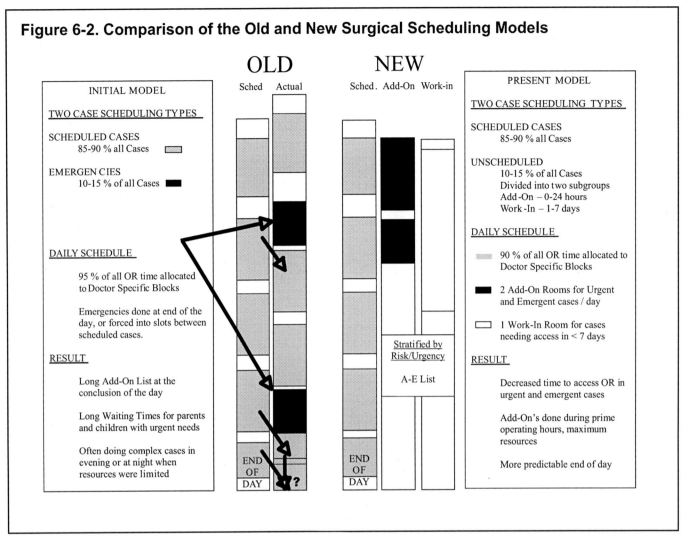

On the basis of the operating room (OR) models, 85% of all OR time was allocated to physician-specific blocks, two add-on rooms were set aside each day for A–E cases, and one room was set aside for work-in cases needing access in less than seven days.

Source: *Cincinnati Children's Hospital Medical Center. Used with permission.*

Although not formally measured, staff satisfaction appeared to improve using this model, as the end of the day was more predictable, emergencies were dealt with in a consistent fashion, and timely access improved staff interactions with families.

Smoothing ICU Demand

A second significant area for improvement of unnatural variability was the scheduling of surgical cases requiring a postoperative stay in the pediatric ICU. Because they represented a need for a limited and resource-intense bed, smoothing of inflow and predictable need allowed better access and planning for ICU services. Although elective surgical cases occupied only 20% to 30% of the pediatric ICU beds, they represented a significant and extremely variable portion of daily admissions and discharges, with significant variations in LOS associated with specific procedures (that is ICU bed turnover). The remainder of the admissions represented patients with multiple trauma or other ED cases

and pediatric medical patients. These streams were most influenced by natural variation because they were not scheduled admissions.

Initial analysis of the elective pediatric ICU surgical population revealed three distinct groups, segmented by their predicted LOS (*see* Table 6-3, page 105). Because many of these admissions required short-term recovery observation and care after elective surgery, it was not surprising that this first group represented the greatest number of patients (61%), and their mean LOS was 1.27 days. The second, smaller group (28%) represented patients with intermediate LOS, occupying a pediatric ICU bed for an average of 3.72 days. The third group, even though they represented a small population numerically (11%), were long-stay patients. This group, which occupied beds for an average of 9.76 days and also had high variability in occupancy, proved to have the most significant impact on pediatric ICU flow. As can be seen in Figure

Chapter 6: *Cincinnati Children's Hospital Medical Center: Redesigning Perioperative Flow Using Operations Management Tools to Improve Access and Safety*

105

Figure 6-3. Add-on Access to Operating Room (OR) Within Accepted Time Frame: Wait Time for A Cases, July 2006–April 2009

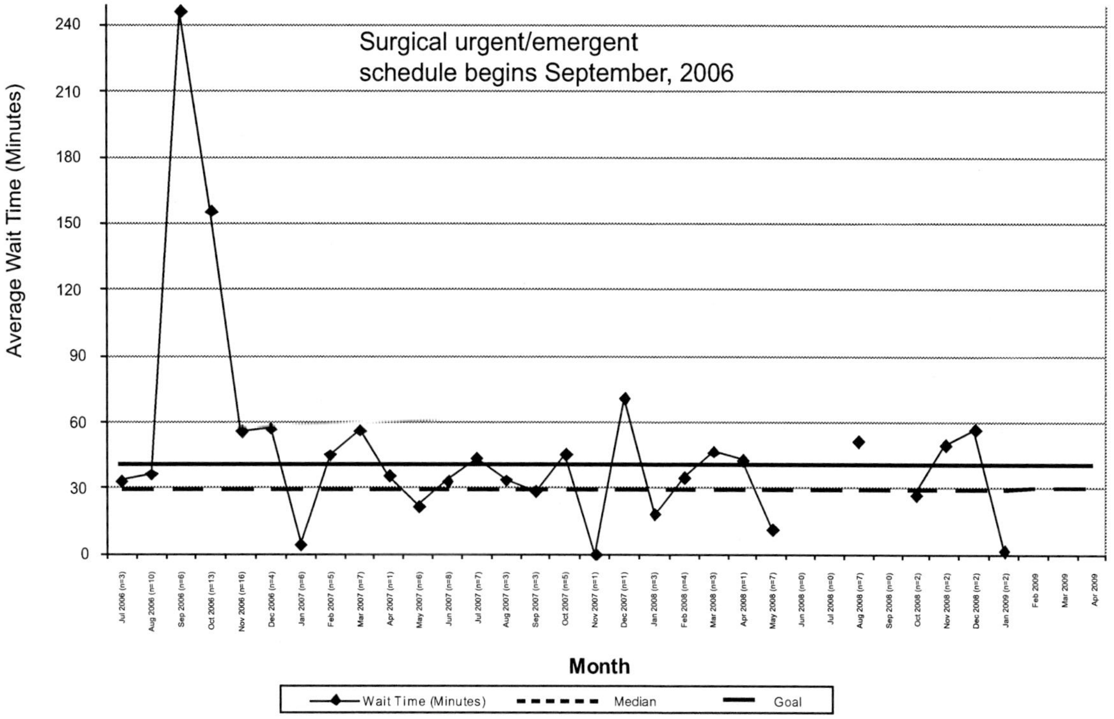

As a result of the redesign, weekday waiting times decreased by 28%, despite a 24% increase in case volume.

Source: *Cincinnati Children's Hospital Medical Center. Used with permission.*

Table 6-3. Case Statistics by Category

Category	Total ICU Days	Case Counts	Average Length of Stay
Short	224.47	177 (61%)	1.27 (27%)
Medium	304.74	82 (28%)	3.72 (37%)
Long	302.56	31 (11%)	9.76 (36%)
Total	831.78	290	2.87

Source: Cincinnati Children's Hospital Medical Center. Used with permission.

6-4 (page 106), the long-stay patients had a greater bed occupancy impact than did the much more numerous short-stay patients. On the basis of an analysis of these groups, a numeric cap was defined to force spread and smoothing at the time of scheduling (*see* Figure 6-5, page 107). This capping model was initially established at five cases per day but has changed as pediatric ICU capacity has varied. Analysis of the long-stay cases showed them, in majority, to be related to complex airway reconstructions. The impact of these long-stay cases on pediatric ICU bed turnover was smoothed by an internal monitor in otolaryngology scheduling, where projected LOS was used to limit the number of occupied pediatric ICU beds for elective airway reconstructions to three on any given day. This spaced the elective long cases, decreasing their prolonged impact on pediatric ICU when excessive numbers were done in clusters. It is important to note that case volume and projected growth were anticipated and accommodated in these

Figure 6-4. Distribution of Procedure Volumes and Pediatric ICU (PICU) Average Length of Stay (ALOS)

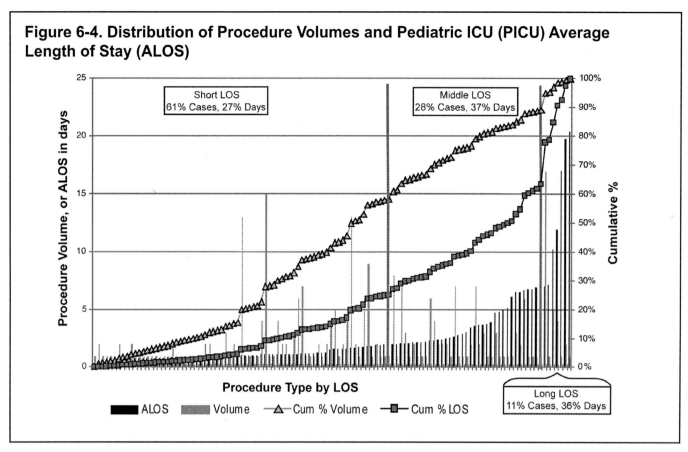

These data, collected during a four-month period, indicate that the long-stay patients had a greater bed occupancy impact than the much more numerous short-stay patients. Each data point represents a separate patient on the x axis reviewed from the database of ICU admissions. *Cum,* cumulative.

Source: *Cincinnati Children's Hospital Medical Center. Used with permission.*

smoothing predictions. As a consequence, there has been no limitation of overall access and no cap on overall case volume. In fact, a 7% growth in operative volume has occurred throughout this time.

A benefit of elective case smoothing has been a decrease in the need to divert overflow cases into other ICU beds, primarily the cardiac pediatric ICU. Although this method is still used on occasion to accommodate demand, it is now uncommon (*see* Figure 6-6, page 108). In addition, the postanesthesia care unit was often used as a substitute overflow pediatric ICU. Because this unit does not have staff with the same level of experience as the pediatric ICU and the nurse–patient ratios are not as high, its interchangeability with the pediatric ICU was limited. Since decreasing the variation in scheduling, use of the postanesthesia care unit has been unnecessary, ensuring that all patients are in suitable ICU environments.

Before implementing these operations management strategies, cases were cancelled when ICU resources were not available for

postoperative management. The policy at Cincinnati Children's is to never begin a case requiring ICU care if this resource is not predictably available. In the absence of the smoothing efforts, periodic high-volume influxes of elective patients, especially long-stay patients, would have a significant and long-standing impact on the availability of beds. Case cancellations have occurred a total of 10 times on 5 separate days in the past 2 years. When a rare cancellation is necessary, the service affected is rotated, and every effort is made to ensure that the case is rescheduled and completed within 24 hours.

Comments from Clinicians

After implementation, partners at the Management Variability Program asked clinicians a series of questions about setting aside ORs for add-on cases. A representative selection of their comments, which were almost uniformly positive, is shown in Table 6-4 (*see* page 109). The respondents felt that the changes had improved satisfaction for parents, their colleagues, and other OR professionals.

Chapter 6: *Cincinnati Children's Hospital Medical Center: Redesigning Perioperative Flow Using Operations Management Tools to Improve Access and Safety*

107

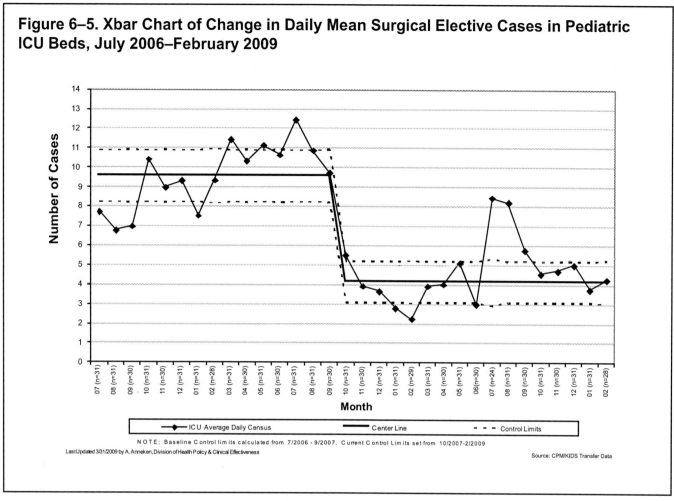

Figure 6–5. Xbar Chart of Change in Daily Mean Surgical Elective Cases in Pediatric ICU Beds, July 2006–February 2009

The xbar chart shows variability around the mean, so that the decrease, as shown, is equivalent to decreased variability of the process. The numeric cap was used to limit the peaks, which effectively smooths flow by spreading the cases to other, less-filled, days. This mechanism is in place as the case is booked, so a case cannot be booked on a day when the cap on elective cases is reached, and another day must be picked. Emergencies are still done as needed.

Source: *Cincinnati Children's Hospital Medical Center. Used with permission.*

Discussion

Efforts at Cincinnati Children's highlight the contrasting approaches of building more resources (ICU beds, ORs) versus using operations management techniques to improve flow, with a strategy to grow programs and expand volume. Establishing improvement as the core business strategy is important to inspire and sustain improvement efforts throughout the organization.[13–15] In the past, most organizations responded to overcrowding, diversions, and delays with expensive rebuilding programs, creating more resources rather than improving utilization of existing resources. In this economically sensitive time, a strategy of building for success is doomed to failure. A more successful approach is to build resources and strategies to maximize their utilization and efficiency.

A health care system is not a machine; rather, it functions as a complex adaptive system.[16–18] It is complex because of the many interconnections between its many parts (for example, ORs, ICUs, ED, laboratories, nurses, physicians, specialists, health plans, accreditors, regulators). It is adaptive in that it is composed of people who can change their behavior. Like ecosystems, complex adaptive systems evolve, adapt, and respond. However, the way individuals in a complex adaptive system act and how that action changes the context for others is not always predictable or linear.[17–19]

Addressing flow is a difficult task because there are so many participants, with different perspectives and priorities. Flow streams need to be carefully identified, quantified, and managed. Flow decisions are important to good patient care and cannot occur by accident. Flow is a complex interaction between many

Figure 6-6. Daily Mean Surgical Elective Cases in the Cardiac ICU, November 2007–June 2009

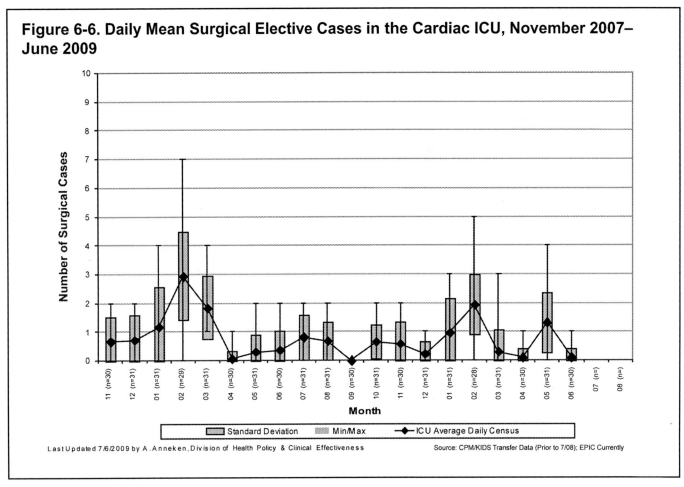

Cardiac ICU stays are considered diversions; patients should be placed in the pediatric ICU.

Source: *Cincinnati Children's Hospital Medical Center. Used with permission.*

different factors in complex environments. The majority of unpredictable factors in flow are determined by the care providers. The use of appropriate operations management techniques allows health care providers to supply improved patient care, timely access to limited services, and patient-centered intervention using available resources by decreasing artificial, often provider-directed, variability.

The keys to improving flow at Cincinnati Children's included outstanding data and sound mathematical models to optimize patient care. The models allowed experimentation with the system variables "outside" the system. Clinicians were actively involved in project planning and the classification of cases according to the A–E categories. Ensuring surgeons that their time in the OR would not be limited was important to gain their support. The revised surgical scheduling system linked the surgical case to the need for an ICU bed, allowing for improved planning and flow in the pediatric ICU. The morning huddle allowed the varied participants to be aware of the daily status and to anticipate the needs for the next day. Throughout the entire project,

Cincinnati Children's was supported by strong leadership committed to solve day-to-day issues as they arose and keep the organization focused on the long-term goals.

This project also resulted in a culture change in the surgical provider environment, improving mutual accountability, open communication, and team mentality. In the old system, access was primarily driven by the chronology of case booking—a first-come, first-served system. Although case urgency was considered, the time of case booking was the primary determinant in most instances. This system fostered the surgeon behavior of working urgent cases into the middle of the elective OR schedule, displacing elective cases into the later day and, often, the evening. Patient satisfaction and operative day prediction for staffing were compromised. In contrast, in the urgency-based add-on system, access is urgency directed and time-goal driven. This has improved not only timely access for all patients but has also decreased ED delays awaiting OR access and ensured urgent access to the most significantly endangered patients (classification A).

Chapter 6: *Cincinnati Children's Hospital Medical Center: Redesigning Perioperative Flow Using Operations Management Tools to Improve Access and Safety*

109

Table 6-4. Comments from Clinicians*

---

1. Did you experience any improvement (or other changes) in your work due to the recent creation of specific rooms for add-on cases? If yes, what kind of improvement?

"This is the best thing for ortho since I have been here. With the additional add-on rooms and our new first available surgeon policy, we almost always get our add-ons done in the early AM, which makes our families very happy. The weekends are unbelievably good. We get our case done early, and patients don't have to wait NPO until the evenings to have their surgery. This has made call much less stressful for my surgeons and myself. The OR is now happy to let us do our add-on cases on weekends, and the hostility has been virtually eliminated." — *Orthopedic surgeon, division director*

"Improved access, less waiting time on weekends and on the weekdays." — *Pediatric surgeon, attending*

"I have only had two opportunities to appreciate the impact of this change. In one instance, no add-on room was available, and both patients had to wait 4 hours until an OR was available. In the other instance, a room was available within 30 minutes." — *Pediatric surgeon, attending*

"I feel there is an improvement in our time and efficiency when assigning staff. We assign add-on staff the day before, instead of 'pulling' staff from rooms. Knowing that we are opening 2 rooms in the morning is easier and more predictable." — *OR nurse*

---

2. Is it easier to schedule add-on cases now, compared to the old system? If yes, what specifically is easier?

"Yes. Less delay, less haggling to get cases done." — *General/thoracic surgeon, attending*

"I believe that we are better able to serve the add-on patients now. There are not as many days when there are 12 add-ons at 6:15 in the morning." — *OR nurse*

---

3. Have your add-on patients been able to have their surgeries more quickly than before the changes? If yes, how do you think it influences the quality of care?

"Definitely. I think emergency cases now happen in an urgent manner — rather than waiting hours for an OR." — *General/thoracic surgeon, attending*

"Add-on patients have been able to get surgery earlier in the day than before. There are fewer complaints about being hungry all day." — *Orthopedic surgeon, attending*

"The family satisfaction with their experience is better than it used to be." — *ENT surgeon, attending*

---

4. Do you think that the change has influenced parents' satisfaction with their child's care (e.g., as a result of a decreased waiting time for surgery)?

"We have not had anywhere near the patient complaints or physician complaints. Physician and family satisfaction has skyrocketed. Ask our ortho nurse specialist how much time she had to spend comforting patients and families during the prior all-day waiting process." — *Orthopedic surgeon, division director*

"Yes — more efficient OR means patients get to surgery in a more timely fashion." — *General/thoracic surgeon, attending*

"As a general rule, I believe the new system is satisfying most families and patients." — *OR nurse*

---

5. What impact have these changes had on your or your colleagues' level of satisfaction with OR operations?

"Less stress, delay, frustration." — *General/thoracic surgeon, attending*

"More operations during the day — instead of night time — seems well received so far." — *Orthopedic surgeon, attending*

(continued on page 110)

Source: Cincinnati Children's Hospital Medical Center. Used with permission.

Table 6-4. *(continued from page 109)*

> "Getting the add-on list done during the day has been nice." — *ENT surgeon, attending*
>
> "The sometimes extreme pressure we felt from dissatisfied surgeons and/or families has seemed to greatly decrease. We have more options now. Earlier, there was nowhere to go with cases!" — *OR nurse*
>
> **6. What do you think has been the impact of these changes on other OR professionals (i.e., nurses, anesthesiologists)?**
>
> "Anesthesia team more willing to do cases knowing we have guidelines — not dependent on surgeon availability or convenience (seems to have been major gripe)." — *Orthopedic surgeon, attending*
>
> "As a general observation, nursing staff 'on call' are not staying as late due to add-ons remaining at change of shift." — *OR nurse*
>
> **7. Are there any other comments you would like to make about the creation of the add-on rooms?**
>
> "Let's fine-tune it—but overall a big step in the right direction." — *Orthopedic surgeon, attending*
>
> "Don't stop here." — *ENT surgeon, attending*
>
> "Life just seems to be significantly more peaceful at the front desk since the creation of the add-on rooms. This says to me that for the most part, we have surgeons, families, and other staff who are more content. There are always 'those days' that are not good, but they seem fewer and fewer as time goes on." — *OR nurse*
>
> * NPO, nothing by mouth; OR, operating room; ENT, ear, nose, and throat.

Although this redesigned system required cooperation and availability of the surgeons, it has also given them and their patients better utilization and access, thus increasing their buy-in. The operative schedule has become more reliable for anesthesia and nursing, which allows them to anticipate and more often meet end-of-the day predictions. For patients and families, because the surgical schedule is more likely to be followed, they have less anxiety, and their stay is more predictable.

As a consequence of smoothing elective surgical cases, in the ICU Cincinnati Children's observed a near elimination of placement of ICU patients into long-term recovery room beds because of lack of ICU availability (inappropriate holds), a decreased need for diversion of postoperative patients to a secondary unit for care because of ICU bed unavailability (inappropriate diversions), a near elimination of cancelled elective surgical cases because of a lack of postoperative ICU beds, and a planned increase in operative volume without the need to construct additional ICU beds.

Efforts at inflow case smoothing can only be successful when predictable ICU outflow to the correct inpatient unit is available. To match the upcoming transfer bed requirements from the pediatric ICU with preferred outflow inpatient units, Cincinnati Children's implemented a system to predict future pediatric ICU transfer and receiving inpatient floor bed availability. An internally built pediatric ICU discharge and floor discharge prediction computer model allows the use of demand-capacity matching to improve this step. Predicted pediatric ICU discharges for the next day are used to construct a bed plan that reserves needed bed resources when specific inpatient care units are needed, such as airway management, postcardiac surgery, and transplantation. Expansion of this system for demand-capacity matching on a hospitalwide basis is currently under way.

Except for the collection of baseline data, development and implementation of this model was not resource intense. Cincinnati Children's assembled an initial team to structure the urgent/emergent stream separation and construct the necessary case lists (Table 6-1). Postanalysis implementation and ongoing management have been absorbed into the daily work of the perioperative leadership and staff. Since this project began, two system analysts have received training in simulation modeling to support future work.

Modern OR construction cost is rarely less than $800,000 and can regularly reach $2 million.[13] Building more complex facilities, as are needed for cardiac surgery, transplants, and neurosurgery, may double this cost. The business case for better utilization is apparent. This is further strengthened in an urban, land-locked facility such as Cincinnati Children's, where available physical

Chapter 6: *Cincinnati Children's Hospital Medical Center: Redesigning Perioperative Flow Using Operations Management Tools to Improve Access and Safety*

111

space for future ORs is very limited. Since 2006, when the redesign of perioperative flow management was initiated to the end of fiscal year 2009 (June 2008), revenues (total dollars) have increased by 34%; overtime dollars as a percentage of total dollars has decreased by 26% (by 6% in 2007–2008, 20% in 2008–2009), and overtime hours as a percentage of total hours have decreased by 31% (10.2% and 20.6%). Improvements in efficiency have boosted our capacity by the equivalent of a $100 million, 100-bed expansion and increased income from treatment of patients by even more.[20]

Before undertaking this initiative, Cincinnati Children's did not appreciate the complexity of the perioperative system, or the potential for improvement. Staff felt that they were just hostages to the emergency nature of the work and, so, that was their life. However, the result has been a more proactive improvement of care for patients and better staff satisfaction. Surgeon schedule flexibility has been the greatest barrier to change, stressing the system and limiting its growth. The additional responsibilities of surgeons can conflict with the need for availability. Also, services with a limited number of providers do not always have someone free to do an urgent case immediately. However, they still benefit from the system, which "cleans up" the other add-on cases so that the more infrequent users do not come into a very full schedule when they need access or when a small service provider needs access. Everyone benefits from the common good.

Identifying the surgical case mix was critical to understanding urgency equation and needs. The need for complete and accurate data when building this model cannot be overstressed. Correct allocation of resources and acceptable postimplementation use are based on correct predictions of need. These predictions cannot be accurately made if the data constructing the model are inaccurate or incomplete. Good data result in good models, and good models encourage acceptance of change.

The next steps at Cincinnati Children's are all in the inpatient area, matching capacity to demand to maximize bed usage, and in the elective schedule, identifying opportunities to further smooth the elective case mix to allow inpatient capacity to meet demand match without decreasing caseloads. The goal is a redistribution of case volume, not a restriction of case volume.

Better and timely access when care is needed is always better than waiting and compromising. Smoothing care streams has allowed patients to be placed on the most appropriate unit so they can receive the specialty nursing care they need. The concentration of similar patients on a unit also allows optimization of evidence-based care plans. The results at Cincinnati Children's show that better care and safer care do not necessarily mean care that is more expensive. It just requires a better use of resources.

The authors thank Lloyd C. Friend, Kahne M. Springborn, and John Rugg for their help in completing this project.

References

1. Institute for Healthcare Improvement: *Optimizing Patient Flow: Moving Patients Smoothly Through Acute Care Settings.* IHI Innovation Series white paper. Boston: Institute for Healthcare Improvement; 2003. (available on www.IHI.org; accessed Sep.10, 2009).

2. Weissman J.S., et al.: Hospital workload and adverse events. *Med Care* 45:448–455, May 2007.

3. Tibby S.M., et al.: Adverse events in a paediatric intensive care unit: Relationship to workload. *Intensive Care Med* 30:1160–1166, Jun. 2004.

4. Richardson D.B.: Increase in patient mortality at 10 days associated with emergency overcrowding. *Med J Aust* 184:213–216, Mar. 6, 2006.

5. Sprivulis P.C., et al.: The association between hospital overcrowding and mortality among patients admitted via Western Australian emergency departments. *Med J Aust* 184:208–212, Mar. 6, 2006.

6. Britto M.T., et al.: Cincinnati Children's Hospital Medical Center: Transforming care for children and families. *Jt Comm J Qual Patient Saf* 32:541–548, Oct. 2006.

7. Berwick D.M.: A user's manual for the IOM's "Quality Chasm" report. *Health Aff (Millwood)* 21:80–90, May–Jun. 2002.

8. Litvak E., Long M.C.: Cost and quality under managed care: Irreconcilable differences? *Am J Manag Care* 6:305–312, Mar. 2000.

9. McManus M.L., et al.: Variability in surgical caseload and access to intensive care services. *Anesthesiology* 98:1491–1496, Jun. 2003.

10. Litvak E., et al.: Managing unnecessary variability in patient demand to reduce nursing stress and improve patient safety. *Jt Comm J Qual Patient Saf* 31:330–338, Jun. 2005.

11. Luria J.W., et al.: Reliability science and patient safety. *Pediatr Clin North Am* 53:1121–1133, Dec. 2006.

12. Ryckman F.C., et al.: Redesigning intensive care unit flow using variability management to improve access and safety. *Jt Comm J Qual Patient Saf* 35:535–543, Nov. 2009.

13. Homer C., Child Health Business Case Working Group: Exploring the business case for improving the quality of health care for children. *Health Aff (Millwood)* 23:159–166, Jul.–Aug. 2004.

14. Leatherman S., et al.: The business case for quality: Case studies and an analysis. *Health Aff (Millwood)* 22:17–30, Mar.–Apr. 2003.

15. Reiter K.L., et al.: How to develop a business case for quality. *Int J Qual Health Care* 19:50–55, Feb. 2007.

16. McDaniel R.R., Jr., Lanham H.J., Anderson R.A.: Implications of complex adaptive systems theory for the design of research on health care organizations. *Health Care Manage Rev* 34:191–199, Apr.–Jun. 2009.

17. Plsek P.E., Greenhalgh T.: The challenge of complexity in health care. *BMJ* 323:625–628, Sep. 2001.

18. Plsek P.E., Wilson T.: Complexity, leadership, and management in healthcare organizations. *BMJ* 323:746–749, Sep. 2001.

19. Bentley F., Chopra M., Price G.: *Future of the Operating Room: Strategic Forecast and Investment Blueprint.* Washington, DC: Health Care Advisory Board, 2006.

20. Allen S.: No waiting: A simple prescription that could dramatically improve hospitals—And American health. *Boston Globe,* Aug. 30, 2009. http://www.boston.com/bostonglobe/ideas/articles/2009/08/30/a_simple_change_could_dramatically_improve_hospitals_ndash_and_american_health_care/?page=full (accessed Sep.10, 2009).

Chapter 7

Kaiser Permanente Southern California, Kaiser Foundation Hospital in Anaheim: Optimizing Patient Flow

Judy Kibler, R.N.; M.Ed.; Marlean Free, Ph.D.; Maria Lee, Ph.D., M.B.A.; Kirk Rinella, M.B.A., R.C.P.; Judy White; Ed Ellison, M.D.; Julie Miller-Phipps; Lisa Schilling, R.N., M.P.H.

Founded in 1945, Kaiser Permanente (KP) is a nonprofit health plan and delivery system headquartered in Oakland, California. KP serves 8.7 million members in nine states and the District of Columbia. Today, it encompasses the nonprofit Kaiser Foundation Health Plan, Inc., Kaiser Foundation Hospitals and their subsidiaries, and the for-profit Permanente Medical Groups. KP is divided into eight regions across the United States, each with its own regional administrative systems and medical group administration. KP is a highly unionized organization, with one of the largest labor and management partnerships of its kind in health care. Staff and physician numbers include approximately 156,000 technical, administrative, and clerical employees and caregivers, as well as 13,000 physicians representing all specialties.

KP's Southern California region employs more than 55,000 technical and clerical employees and caregivers and more than 6,000 physicians. Together they provide health care services to 3.3 million members at the Southern California region's 12 medical centers and more than 130 medical offices.

The KP-wide performance improvement system includes a network of more than 300 staff "trained as experts"—improvement advisers (IAs), who work with facility operations teams to redesign processes from the patient's point of view. The IAs and a number of other key players—from frontline workers to top executives—receive specialized training through a fellowship-like program called the Improvement Institute. This allows the organization to focus on capability and results rather than methods of improvement. Twelve experts in systems thinking and improvement methods deployed to assist IAs, teams, and operational leaders understand system-level priorities, determine drivers of performance, and establish a sequence plan for portfolios of improvement necessary to improve system performance.

Kaiser Foundation Hospital Anaheim

The Kaiser Foundation Hospital Anaheim (Anaheim) is a full-service medical facility in Anaheim, Orange County, California. It is licensed for 200 beds and has 176 beds operational, with approximately 89% occupancy. Kaiser Permanente Orange County serves approximately 390,000 members through a network of more than 5,200 employees and 650 physicians, 2 hospitals, and 19 medical office facilities.

Identifying the Problem

Two problems have complicated systemwide changes in health care in general and patient flow at Anaheim in particular. First, every division and unit measures its own performance with a variety of data, but it is much more difficult and unusual to track cross-functional activities to determine how well the system as a whole is faring. This leads to managing to peaks in census and acuity but not necessarily managing to reduce variation. As a result, patients experience waits, delays, and little predictability in their progress through the health care delivery system. Second, most efforts at health care improvement have been driven from the top down. All too often, the frontline people who do the work have not been consulted. This means that sometimes the wrong problem is solved, or a "fix" is put on top of day-to-day work, thus making it more complicated for day-to-day operations to sustain improvement.

Efforts to improve patient flow at Anaheim began in 2004 in this fashion. Cross-functional management teams assessed bed turnover and worked with departments such as the emergency department (ED), the medical/surgical unit, and the ICU in an attempt to improve the various factors affecting bed turnover, such as admitting procedures, discharge processes, and bed readiness. For example, the hospital had hired a bed utilization leader and instituted interdisciplinary bed huddles, but progress was mixed; improvement was neither sufficient nor sustained.

In January 2008, "divert" hours (when the hospital is closed to emergency and new patients) were very high—302 for the month. "Boarder" hours—how long patients must wait in the ED—were also high, at 55 per month. In addition, 1.8% of patients left without being seen (LWBS)—also an unacceptably high number—and complaints from patients about having to wait in the ED were numerous.

Management wanted to look at patient flow differently. The perception was that backups in the ICU were causing the problem. However, the systemwide flow analysis showed that the ICU admission process was not the bottleneck. Although the admit process time (APT)—the time it takes to admit patients from the ED to the appropriate department—was sometimes long, as much as 5.5 hours, it was the patient transfer process that was slow, meaning that beds were often not available when there was demand from patients waiting in the ED.

Patient flow had been assessed previously with several measures. Patient surveys measured complaints about delays in care. Admit process time was measured, but there was no tracking of actual transfer time to specific departments, just a "hunch" that certain transfer times were long. Anaheim also tracked average peak discharge time, which, in early 2008, was between 4 P.M. (16:00) and 5 P.M. (17:00), which was not optimal because of change-of-shift times and working hours. In addition, nurses' wait with the patients, and thus overtime charges, were high as nurses waited past their shift times for patients to be discharged late in the day.

Tension between the various departments was exacerbated because the other departments assumed that the patient flow backlog was originating in the ICU, and blaming other departments for problems became the standard. Patients complained about the long delay in being processed, and the dissatisfaction showed up in both complaints filed and the percentage of patients who LWBS.

A New Start

In 2006, as part of a partnership with the Institute for Healthcare Improvement (IHI), KP began an effort to help its Southern California medical centers address patient flow in a thoroughgoing, systemwide approach. In late 2007, KP began implementing a performance improvement operating system that was designed to assist operational executives in applying execution modeling and improvement methodologies to create and sustain improvement. As one of the initial KP sites, the executive team at Anaheim had focused on a key strategic goal: *Orange County patients would be cared for in KP Orange County facilities (rather than being cared for elsewhere)*. The planned approach would be to focus on first reducing variation and waste to improve predictability and then matching demand for resources with the capacity to provide resources in beds and staffing.

An additional goal was to develop effective practices that could be shared between the service area's medical centers and across the entire organization so that the whole system could improve. This would be achieved by identifying all the drivers of performance in throughput, the areas that, if optimally managed, would provide better flow through the system. A next step would be to identify a portfolio of patient flow projects that, if sequentially implemented, would produce the desired outcome—that is, ensuring that Anaheim could care for its own members at this facility without the need to use outside hospital services.

Anaheim's leadership team decided to sponsor the program, and an interdisciplinary throughput team was formed (with frontline staff included for the first time; *see* Table 7-1, page 115), reporting to the utilization management committee. However, after the first project team was created later that year, the executive sponsors realized the need for a specific oversight committee. The

Table 7-1. Members of the Interdisciplinary Frontline Teams for Hospital Patient Flow*

- Bed utilization nurse (BUN)

- Bed utilization director

- Ward clerks

- Staff nurses

- Environmental services supervisor

- Emergency department improvement advisor

- Emergency department team co-lead (charge nurse)

- Transfer/discharge improvement advisor

- Transfer/discharge team co-leads (assistant department administrator and charge nurse)

- Senior data consultant

- Discharge planner/case manager

- Continuing care service-line leader

- Inpatient service-line leader

- Ambulatory care service-line leader

- Surgical services service-line leader

- Primary care service-line leader

- Physician champions

Source: Kaiser Foundation Hospital Anaheim. Used with permission.

performance improvement strategic oversight committee—a dedicated group that would to provide each team with a focused review of its progress, lessons learned, and barriers encountered—was formed, with a portfolio of eight projects related to improving patient flow at Anaheim. The goals and responsibilities of the oversight committee were as follows:

■ Lead implementation of the performance improvement projects and system, as well as oversight and learning at Anaheim and Irvine Medical Center (also part of Orange County)

■ Oversee the progress of the portfolio of projects in the context of the entire organization's operations

■ Review and approve the business case for specific projects

■ Ensure the communication and spread of learning throughout the organization

■ Develop the capacity to sustain improvement gains

The portfolio of projects was determined by Anaheim's executive leaders and a dedicated full-time IA. The IA, responsible for the overall progress of a multiyear strategy to improve flow, facilitated the transfer/discharge team discussions and decision making, supported/coached the part-time IAs, developed the necessary infrastructure, coordinated staff training, and communicated program progress to leaders regionally and nationally.

The work began with a multiday workshop in March 2008 to identify the systems drivers and map the entire patient flow process. To ensure that whole-system changes were implemented, drivers of performance in throughput were identified (*see* Figure 7-1, page 116), and eight projects were scoped. The projects within the overall flow portfolio were scoped into 90- to 120-day efforts that engaged cross-functional teams, with a distinct team created for each project. The first three projects were as follows: an ICU transfer to floor project initiated in March 2008, a discharge from floor to home or skilled nursing facility project initiated in October 2008, and an ED to floor admit process time project initiated in October 2008.

The interdisciplinary nature of the teams proved to be important, but communication early on was an issue, given the rapid pace of daily work in a hospital. Therefore, bed huddles were increased to three per day, with an emphasis on huddling at the change in shift so that cross-department staff leads were involved. This allowed for predictability in patient volumes and movement, along with deploying staffing as demand warranted throughout a given period of time.

Measuring Patient Flow

The throughput teams realized that although opportunities existed to streamline the transfer processes, the major barrier was bed availability to the floor. The importance of knowing how the entire system functions became apparent, together with the need to ensure that improvement in one area did not cause problems in another.

One of the most significant initial problems was that, at first, Anaheim had no good agreed-on metrics for transfer time. Therefore, the initial work of the teams was focused on creating metrics to monitor improvement (*see* Table 7-2, page 117). In addition, local department data needed to be integrated to (1) better predict seasonal variation in both patient demand for services and patient-acuity patterns and to (2) adopt staffing patterns that responded to such demand rather than staffing for the average daily census. For example, KP opened a second hospital, KP Irvine, in the service area in May 2008, and it had

Figure 7-1. Drivers of Effective Flow, Anaheim Medical Center

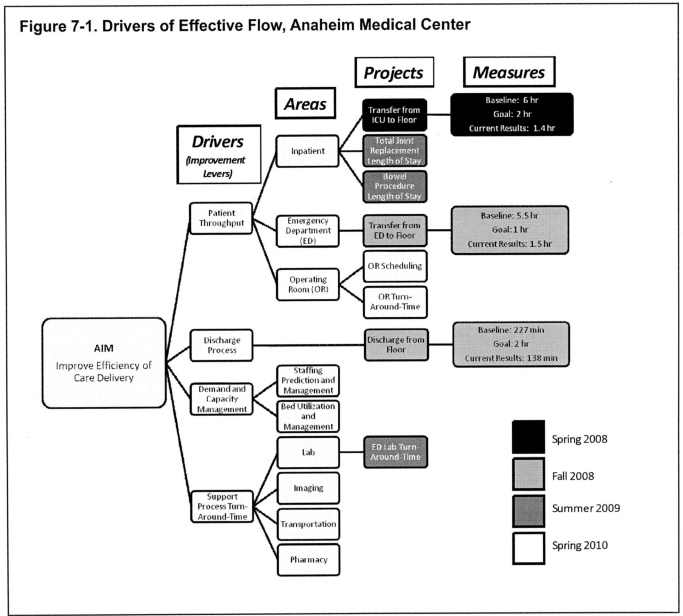

This figure shows the primary levers that drive improvement in throughput (key functional areas of work) and the sequence of projects in the overall flow portfolio. Measures are identified for completed projects as of August 2009. The black boxes relate to the Transfer Time When Bed Given from the ICU to Floor project, initiated in Spring 2008. Light gray projects were initiated in Fall 2008. Dark gray projects were initiated in Summer 2009, and white projects are expected to commence in Spring 2010.

Source: *Kaiser Foundation Hospital Anaheim. Used with permission.*

been planned to reduce Anaheim's demand by 15%. However, right before a local community hospital, Irvine Regional Hospital, closed in January 2009, it mailed leaflets to the public that announced the availability of ED services at Anaheim—resulting in an 11% increase in demand after the initial 15% reduction was realized with the opening of KP Irvine. This situation might have been predicted, and data showing the impact of changes in community availability could have assisted operational leaders to monitoring ED demand and system availability to determine how Anaheim could best address a sudden increase in ED patient volumes.

At first, data for the ICU-to-floor-transfer measures (time physician writes the transfer order, time bed given/assigned, time bed available (clean and ready), time patient left the unit) were manually collected in daily logs by the ICU ward clerks. The data collection process is now automated, and data are collected in real time. For example, an automatic printout documents a transfer order, and a general "new order" list is available through Anaheim's automated KP HealthConnect™ electronic health record (EHR) system. Time stamps in the EHR system enable automated reports that allow day-by-day determination of performance on all the ICU-to-floor transfer metrics. The key metric

Table 7-2. Key Measures of Patient Flow for the Initial Transfer, Discharge, and Emergency Department (ED) Patient Flow Projects, Including Operational Definitions of Calculated Measures, Anaheim Medical Center

Key Transfer Measures	Time Physician Writes Transfer Order
	Time Bed Given (assigned)
	Time Bed Available (bed clean and ready)
	Time Patient Leaves the Unit
	Transfer Time When Bed Available (TWBA=Time Patient Leaves the Unit-Time Bed Available)
	Transfer Time When Bed Given (TWBG=Time Patient Leaves Unit-Time Bed Given)
	Total Transfer Time (=Time Patient Leaves Unit-Time Physician Writes Transfer Order)
	Number of transfer delays (Total Transfer Time when bed available > 1 hour)
Key Discharge Measures	Time Physician Writes Discharge Order
	Time Patient Leaves the Unit
	Discharge Time (=Time Patient Leaves the Unit-Time Physician Writes Discharge Order)
	Percent of Patients for which Discharge Time was > 2 hours
	Average Peak Discharge Time
Key ED Flow Measures	Time Physician Writes Admit Order
	Time Bed Assigned
	Time Patient Leaves the ED
	Admit Process Time (APT=Time Patient Leaves the ED-Time Physician Writes Admit Order)
	Bed Assigned to Out of ED (=Time Patient Leaves the ED-Time Bed Assigned)
	ASQ Survey ED Patient Overall Satisfaction

Source: Kaiser Foundation Hospital Anaheim. Used with permission.

data are shared daily in huddles and are compiled into reports that are subsequently shared (1) weekly among improvement team members; (2) monthly with the oversight team, champions, and service-line leaders; and (3) quarterly with the KP region.

Implementation of Strategies

The patient flow improvement program began in March 2008, with an initial focus (based on the system assessment and macro-process map) on reducing patient transfer time from the ICU to the medical/surgical floor. Although the availability of beds in the ICU was identified as a bottleneck, an integrated systems view (Figure 7-1) revealed a series of issues, including a problem with patient discharge and a need to understand what support function turnaround times needed to be improved to help patients move more efficiently from one department to another. For example, laboratory draws and results turnaround times emerged as contributors to delays in the transfer of ED patients to the floor, reflecting the fact that laboratory results are needed before a decision is made to admit from the ED.

With management oversight and buy-in, the program's multidisciplinary teams—the ICU floor transfer team, the discharge from floor team, and the ED to floor team—met for several days to assess the problem, create process flow maps for the entire end-to-end flow through the hospital and flow from one unit to another (*see* Figure 7-2, page 118, and Figure 7-3, page 119), and identify sources of process variation and opportunities for improvement. For example, the ICU to floor transfer team determined that major sources of variation were inconsistent communication procedures between the physician and the nurse regarding transfer and discharge orders; inconsistent communication between the ward clerk, the bed utilization nurse (BUN), and environmental services (EVS) regarding bed-clean status; and patient transport delays. Areas of waste included waiting for someone to clean a room, waiting for notification that a bed was ready, and waiting for the generation of reports indicating which patients needed to be transferred. Variation and waste reduced the ability of the staff on each unit to predict how quickly a patient would transfer after an order is written.

The three teams established realistic goals and metrics and then determined where to start making changes. At every stage, the people accountable for results were the people doing the work. To ensure sustainability of any intervention, each team managed one set of key measures over time—monitoring variation in performance and coordinating involvement of staff and managers in response to variation in real time.

Figure 7-2. Macroprocess Flow Diagram for Patient Movement from ED/ICU Through Discharge, Anaheim Medical Center

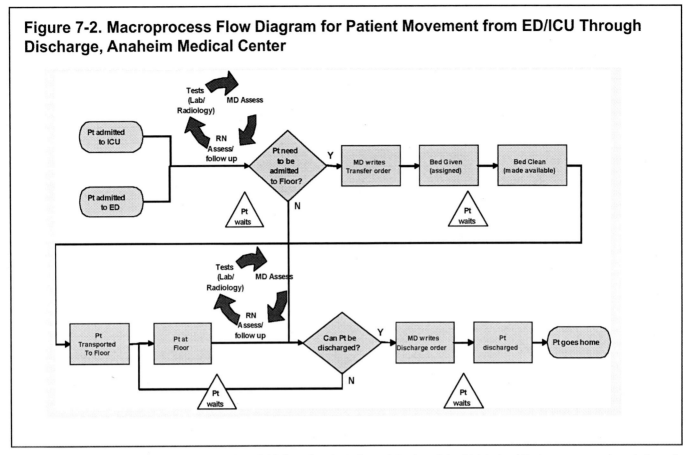

This flow diagram represents a high-level snapshot of the flow of patients through the hospital, which helped the team assess where to focus its improvement efforts and identify the processes that needed to be mapped in more detail (that is, "MD writes transfer order" to "patient at the floor" and "MD writes discharge order" to "patient goes home"). ED, emergency department; MD, medical doctor; Pt, patient; RN, registered nurse.

Source: *Kaiser Foundation Hospital Anaheim. Used with permission.*

Transfer from ICU to Floor Project

There were two distinct goals for this project, initiated in March 2008:

    1. Decrease the transfer time from the ICU to the medical/surgical floors when the bed is given/assigned from six hours to two hours by December 2008.

    2. Transfer patients from the ICU to the medical/surgical floors within one hour of bed assignment by the bed utilization nurse (BUN) by December 2008.

Process Changes. To achieve these goals, several process changes were planned and tested in a 90-day period. These changes were designed to simplify and standardize the transfer process for all shifts:

• *EHR Flag of Patient Ready for Transfer.* The data initially showed that the delay between the physician writing a transfer order to the nurse becoming aware of the order varied from 5 minutes to 20 hours. After the nurse knew that a patient was able to be moved, a bed had to be found—which meant cleaning and

prepping the space. With the move to electronic records, there were no visual cues to alert the nurse that a patient was ready for transfer. Accordingly, an initial change was to create a flag in the EHR to improve the response and decrease variability in the time it took for a staff member to realize that there was an active patient transfer order. Immediately, staff could see a report of all patients ready for transfer from the ICU and in need of beds on a given floor. The team leads compared this list to the rounding predictions with physicians and determined the reliability of their predictions. Through the course of the project, agreement between predicted transfers and actual written orders was maintained at ≥ 90%.

• *Elimination of Separate Team Accountability for Transfer.* The initial change included eliminating using the lift team to perform patient transport, therefore eliminating the wait time associated with this step. It was found that this function was secondary to the life team members' other work. Now ICU staff maintain responsibility for transfer, and ward clerks are trained and prepared to assist with this function.

Figure 7-3. Simplified Process Flow Diagram of Transfer from ICU to Floor and Discharge from Medical/Surgical Floors, Anaheim Medical Center

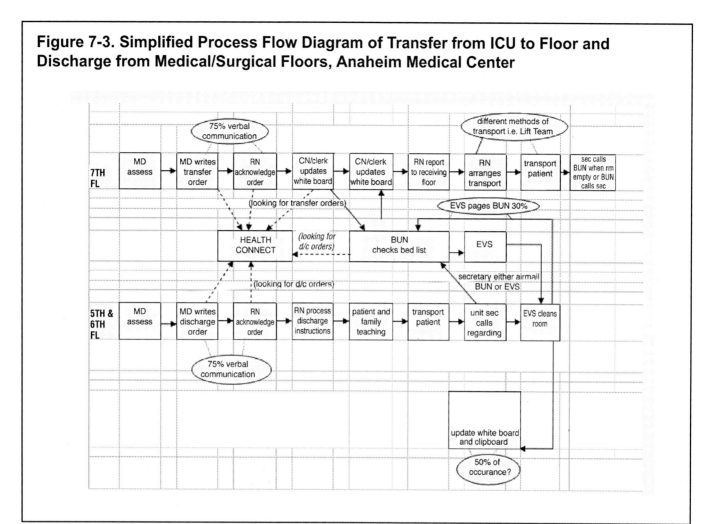

These maps allowed the team to identify sources of variation in the transfer and discharge processes: inconsistent communication procedures between the physician and the nurse regarding transfer and discharge orders; inconsistent communication procedures between the ward clerk, the bed utilization nurse (BUN), and environmental services (EVS) regarding bed status; and transport delays. MD, physician; RN, registered nurse; CN, charge nurse; sec, secretary.

Source: *Kaiser Foundation Hospital Anaheim. Used with permission.*

• *ICU Staff Direct Contact for Room Cleaning and Report.* Handoffs (handovers) between departments and responsiveness also delayed transfer time. To speed the process, the ward clerk was to initiate the cascade after the order was written and the patient was transferred. The ICU ward clerk now calls EVS to have a bed cleaned and notifies the BUN after the bed is ready for admitting a patient to the ICU. Downstream in the process, if the receiving nurse at the floor is unavailable to take the report, the charge nurse now receives the report and maintains accountability for checking the patient into the floor until the floor nurse is available.

• *System to Monitor Performance of Transfer Within One Hour.* After the transfer orders are written and the ward clerk performs the specific tasks outlined, the charge nurse updates the nursing-unit white board with the transfer information. The ward clerk maintains a daily log of all transfers, which includes the key

transfer metrics (Transfer Time When Bed Given [TWBG], Transfer Time When Bed Available [TWBA], and Total Transfer Time). He or she notes the reasons for transfer delays. If the total transfer time is more than one hour, the charge nurse reviews the case and then reviews system issues with the assistant department administrator to determine follow-up action plans. The key transfer metrics are also reported as part of the medical service line's flash report, which is reviewed monthly by the service-line leaders and executives and the performance improvement strategic oversight committee. The key metric monitoring commitments are documented in a "sustainability plan" approved by department administrators and other key players.

Results. As a result of the transfer team's work, TWBG was reduced from an average of six hours (May–November 2008) to 1.4 hours (January–July 2009), as demonstrated in Figure 7-4 (page 120) and Figure 7-5 (page 121). The team was able to

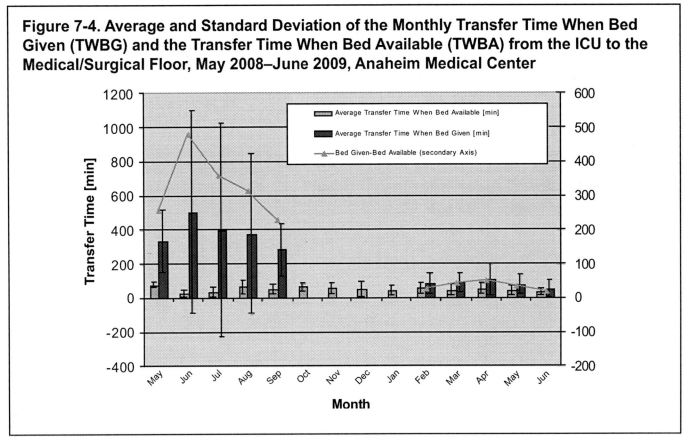

Figure 7-4. Average and Standard Deviation of the Monthly Transfer Time When Bed Given (TWBG) and the Transfer Time When Bed Available (TWBA) from the ICU to the Medical/Surgical Floor, May 2008–June 2009, Anaheim Medical Center

Originally, the variability in TWBG was significant, and the gap between the TWBG and the TWBA was more than 300 hours (light gray line). With the work of the ICU to floor transfer team, the gap between TWBG and TWBA decreased dramatically, translating into much shorter patient wait times.

Source: *Kaiser Foundation Hospital Anaheim. Used with permission.*

dramatically decrease the number of outliers, or individual patients waiting for long periods of time (Figure 7-5), making the transfer process more reliable and predictable and decreasing the occurrence of long wait times once the bed is assigned. This has occurred during a period of time when no significant reduction in patient volumes has occurred. In fact, this performance was maintained during winter months, when patient volumes and acuity commonly increase.

The gap between TWBG and TWBA has also decreased since May 2008 (Figure 7-4), indicating the effect of the streamlining of support processes such as patient transportation and bed cleaning on patient flow. TWBA has been consistently less than 1 hour since January 2009. As of the end of June 2009, the monthly TWBA was 35 minutes. The total transfer time has been reduced from 9.5 hours to less than 7.5 hours and has been maintained at that level, as of August 2009, since April 2009. The dramatic reductions in variability indicate that a more reliable and predictable process for patient transfer has been established.

Transfer delays are now reviewed daily by the charge nurse and the assistant department administrator. The results show that the

majority of patients waiting for more than one hour have been "planned holds" for whom a decision was made by the care team to keep the patient in the ICU and to give the bed to an ED patient, a surgical patient, or an outside (clinic) patient. The second reason for transfers of greater than one hour has been that the clinical condition of the patient changed.

Discharge from Floor Project

The second project initiated in October 2008 was designed to improve the discharge process from the medical/surgical floor. The two goals of this project were as follows:

1. Achieve an average discharge time (the time the patient leaves the unit to the time the physician writes the discharge order) of 2 hours by May 2009 for medical/surgical patients. At the start of project, the average discharge time was 227 minutes.

2. Change the average peak discharge time by 1 hour by May 2009. At the start of project, the average peak discharge time was 4:00 P.M. (16:00).

Process Changes. In analyzing the baseline discharge data, the

Figure 7-5. Weekly ICU to Medical/Surgical Unit Transfer Time When Bed Given (TWBG), May 2008–June 2009, Anaheim Medical Center

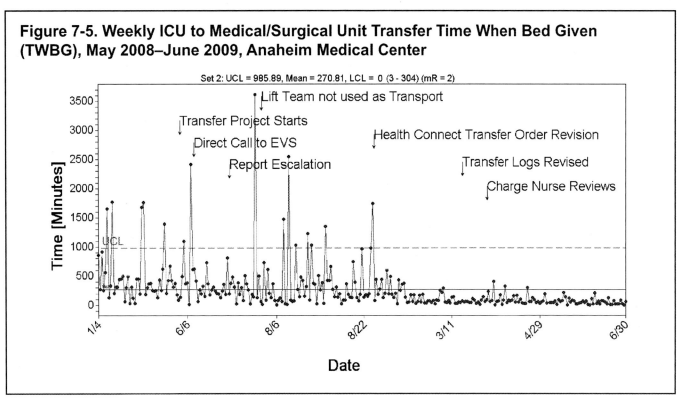

The figure shows the dates of process changes implemented by the team. The transfer time variability and the number of outliers decreased dramatically, particularly after the HealthConnect™ order revision. Mean = 270.81; upper control limit (UCL) = 985.89; lower control limit (LCL) = (not shown).

Source: *Kaiser Foundation Hospital Anaheim. Used with permission.*

discharge team found that the discharges were primarily associated with delays in transporting the patient home, incorrect discharge orders written by the physician staff, and discharge of patients to skilled nurse facilities. All the subsequent process changes, as now described, were focused on addressing these three issues:

• *Planning Discharge with Patients.* Much as it had done with transfers, the staff found that it was able to predict discharges. The team developed a process for the admitting and nursing staffs' early communication with the patient regarding the discharge process, including alternate ride contacts. This change implied a culture shift, particularly for nurses, who were not accustomed to discussing the discharge plan with the patient on admission. The practice was embedded by writing the anticipated discharge date and alternate ride contact information on the patient in-room care board, a white board on which nurses write patient care information. In addition, the patient discharge plan was included as part of the shift-to-shift reports. Furthermore, case managers are now paired with attending physicians on admission so that they can begin discharge planning as early as reasonable.

• *Standardized Discharge Criteria.* Physicians were educated to avoid writing incomplete or incorrect discharge orders.

Physician champions used venues such as the utilization management committee and the department of medicine committee to communicate to their peer group and obtain agreements. The discharge team also worked with physicians to set a standard that all patient discharges did not need to wait for daily rounding. Therefore, practices such as having at least one stable patient discharged before the 10:00 A.M. (10:00) bed huddle helped reinforce the process of discharging when a patient was ready rather than by a set schedule that may not have been best for system flow.

• *Care Management Coordination with Skilled Nursing Facilities.* The care model was changed on the medical/surgical unit to ensure that dedicated case managers could facilitate communication with and access to nursing staff. The pairing of case managers with physicians enabled reductions in the case manager-to-patients ratio and allowed the case manager to see all patients and start the discharge process as soon as the patient's readiness for discharge was known. This eliminated any waiting for support to assist in planning for patient specific discharge or transportation needs.

• *Creation of Unit Bed Huddles.* Unit bed huddles were initiated on every shift to review anticipated discharge needs and to share communication from the interdisciplinary hospitalwide bed huddles, which occurred three times a day, with the staff. The day case manager and the day charge nurse generate the Anticipated Discharge List at the end of their shifts. The evening- and night-shift staff review the list before the hospital and unit bed morning huddles to record updates before discharge plans are finalized for the day. Although there is no formal documentation to determine and show changes in the accuracy in predicting discharges, the discharge team considered the unit bed huddles in conjunction with the Anticipated Discharge List to be key process changes.

• *System to Monitor Performance of Discharge Within Two Hours.* The ward clerks maintain a discharge log at the desk to document the key discharge metrics and reasons for discharge delays. The discharge team co-leads—the charge nurse and the assistant department administrator—review the discharge log and determine follow-up action plans for system-level issues. The service-line leaders and executives and the performance improvement strategic oversight committee review the key discharge metrics on a monthly basis. The key metric monitoring commitments are documented in a Sustainability Plan approved by department administrators and other key players.

Results. As a result of this work, the average discharge time decreased from 217 minutes in the first quarter of 2008 to 162 minutes in the first quarter of 2009, a 26% decrease, as shown in Figure 7-6 (page 123). The average discharge time for June 2009 was 138 minutes. The peak discharge time for May 2009 was 3:06 P.M. (15:06) for medical/surgical floors, and it was 4:00 P.M. (16:00) as of May 2008, reaching the planned goal. Transportation delays remain the most frequent cause for delay in discharge. The charge nurse and/or the assistant department administrator have now been communicating with patients regarding alternative ride contacts, with some success.

Transfer Time from Emergency Department (ED) to Floor

The third project initiated in October 2008 was reducing the ED's APT. The two goals for the ED APT project were as follows:
1. Improve the ED's APT at Anaheim Medical Center from 5.5 hours to within 1 hour by August 2009.
2. Decrease the bed assigned to out of ED time (as defined in Table 7-2) from 61 to 40 minutes by August 2009.

Process Changes. To achieve these goals, the ED team implemented key process changes, as now described:

• *Immediate Notification of Admission Orders.* The ED team implemented a process for texting the admit patient clinical

information to the BUN to ensure that just-in-time bed needs were communicated with management. A service-level agreement was created between the ED and the BUN, in which a response from the BUN is expected within 15 minutes of this initial communication. In addition, the charge nurse in the ED and the patient's ED nurse are paged when the bed is ready at the floor.

• *Standardized Admission Information Tool.* To improve the accuracy of the admission information, the team implemented a form that is provided by the BUN to the admitting unit ward clerk which provides accurate and complete admission information.

• *Reducing Variation Through Accurate Bed Assignments.* The BUN now assigns beds only when they are clean and ready and not when a patient needs one and a floor has a "predicted" transfer or discharge. A bed is not linked to a patient until the bed is clean and ready, which reduces needs to reprioritize patients or revisit the decision should the bed on the floor suddenly not be available because of changes in the patient's condition or other issues.

• *Report When Patient Is Ready.* If the receiving nurse on the floor is unavailable, the ED nurse now goes directly to the receiving unit with the patient and provides the report face to face. Previously, the ED nurse would call the floor repeatedly until the receiving nurse gave the go-ahead by phone for the patient to be brought to the floor. The ED nurse can now make a first call and then a second call within one minute, after which, if the floor nurse cannot be reached, he or she transfers the patient on the gurney into the unit and gives the handoff report directly to the floor nurse at the bedside.

• *Service-Level Agreements: Clarity About "What Good Looks Like."* Several service-level agreements were made so that departments could agree about standards of care, timing, and what good performance consisted of to meet patient needs for care. For example, for the support function of transport, an agreement was established for ED transport to move patients out of the ED within 15 minutes of bed assignment. An agreement was created between EVS and nursing which specified that EVS would provide immediate notification when a bed was ready. In addition, staffing and equipment changes were made to meet demand for services. There is now an EVS cart on each floor with dedicated staff, and EVS staffing is provided during the night. These changes have helped expedite the cleaning of beds and thereby the reduction of transfer times.

Results. These five process changes resulted in a significant reduction in time to admit ED patients to the floor, despite

Figure 7-6. Monthly Average Discharge Time from the Medical/Surgical Floor, January 2008–June 2009, Anaheim Medical Center

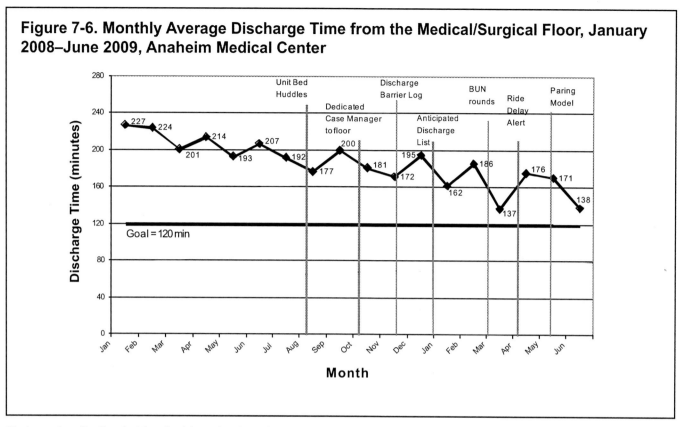

Discharge time (the time that the physician writes the order to the time that the patient leaves the unit) has decreased, contributing to reduction in wait times in the ICU and the emergency department (ED). Annotations reflect the changes implemented by the team. BUN, bed utilization nurse.

Source: *Kaiser Foundation Hospital Anaheim. Used with permission.*

significant fluctuations and increased ED patient volumes over time. The ED's APT decreased by 30% from the first quarter of 2008 to the first quarter of 2009, in spite of seasonal variability. The APT for June 2009 was the lowest monthly value yet observed—1 hour 27 minutes, in comparison with 5 hours 30 minutes in January 2008 and 2 hours 44 minutes in June 2008 (*see* Figure 7-7, page 124). The continuing goal is less than or equal to 1 hour.

The bed assigned to out of ED time decreased from 61 minutes in November 2008 to 38 minutes in April 2009—a 60% decrease. The ED patient overall satisfaction increased from 80% (satisfied) in May 2008 to 90.3% in May 2009, all while patient LWBS rates dropped as volumes increased.

Cumulative Results

Overall, the three patient flow projects at Anaheim have resulted in dramatic improvements in predictability for patient transfer and movement across the system. "We work together as a team now," noted the labor co-lead for the patient flow team (a member of United Nurses Associations of California/Union of Health

Care Professionals), who added, "It used to be that ED got mad at us [for the backup], but there were no beds to give them."

The overall average length of stay (ALOS) decreased slightly—from 3.71 to 3.6—days, and the ALOS variability has also decreased, despite fluctuations in patient volume that resulted from the opening of the KP Irvine facility, the closing of Irvine Regional Hospital, and seasonal effects (*see* Figure 7-8, page 125).

The decreasing trend in daily census before opening the Irvine Medical Center stabilized in July–September 2008 to 135 (15% lower than what it was in January 2008). When the community hospital (Irvine Regional Hospital) closed in January 2009, there was an approximately 11% increase in daily census, resulting in a 4% lower census than the period before the opening of the Irvine Medical Center. These fluctuations are also reflected in the average number of ED visits (*see* Figure 7-9, page 125), with the current volume being greater than changes in hospital bed availability in the community.

The fluctuations in patient volume confound the effects of the implementation of improvements that resulted from the efforts described herein on metrics such as LWBS (*see* Figure 7-10, page

Figure 7-7. Emergency Department (ED) Monthly Admit Process Time (APT), January 2008–June 2009, Anaheim Medical Center

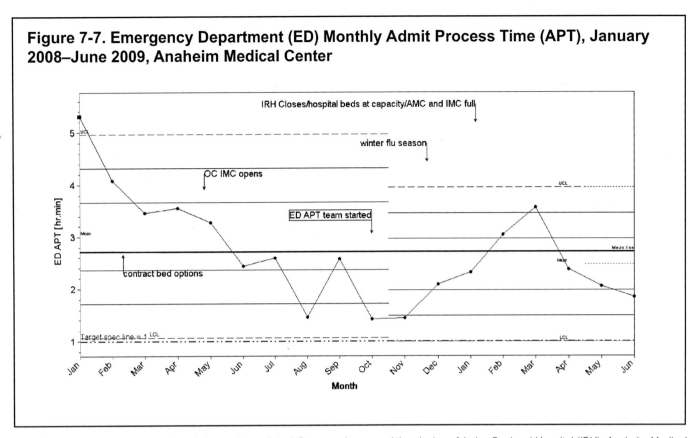

Despite potential special causes in variation such as winter influenza volumes and the closing of Irvine Regional Hospital (IRH), Anaheim Medical Center has reduced its average admit time toward its goal of 1 hour. Mean = 2.47; upper control limit (UCL) = 3.95; lower control limit (LCL) = 0.99.

Source: *Kaiser Foundation Hospital Anaheim. Used with permission.*

126) and ALOS. However, these improvement efforts were a significant contributor to the reduction of variation in system metrics selected to be monitored throughout the program execution. For example, the number of LWBS patients (Figure 7-10) decreased to a record low after January 2009, despite increases in patient volumes reflecting the closure of Irvine Regional Hospital. The monthly ALOS shows decreased variation, regardless of these volume fluctuations (Figure 7-8).

The reduced variation in transfer and discharge times contributed to improved predictability of bed availability and nursing overtime; overtime was reduced by 12% between March 2008 and March 2009. Approximately $800,000 in annual direct and indirect costs and revenue capture was realized by meeting patient and member demand for care and services while maintaining patient volumes and managing seasonal fluctuations in patient acuity. Patient satisfaction scores have improved, reflecting the more efficient flow of patients through the hospital and earlier discharges.

Discussion

Overall, Anaheim Medical Center has achieved its first major goal of improving flow through the hospital—reducing variation in

time for transfer through the system and discharge to home or outside facilities. Reducing the time it takes to admit patients from the ED appears to have enabled Anaheim to manage large fluctuations in patient volumes and meet the needs for beds in the ICU and medical/surgical units while reducing overtime use among nursing staff in the ICU. Furthermore, staff satisfaction has been positively affected as a corollary to the improvement implementations. Interestingly, reduction in process variability is considered in the literature as a significant contributor to the reduction in staff stress and improvement in staff satisfaction.[1]

Kosnik identified five key components of demand capacity management: ability to communicate across silos in a hospital, intradepartmental collaboration, the ability to standardize "best" practices, empowerment of staff, and creation of institutional memory.[2] The most powerful process changes that the Anaheim patient flow teams implemented, such as use of bed huddles and creation of cross-departmental service-level agreements, embrace these elements and enable the process changes to be both repeatable and sustainable.

One of the most critical successes at Anaheim has been the dual focus on improvements at the system and frontline levels. All too

Figure 7-8. Anaheim Medical Center Average Length of Stay (ALOS), January 2008–May 2009

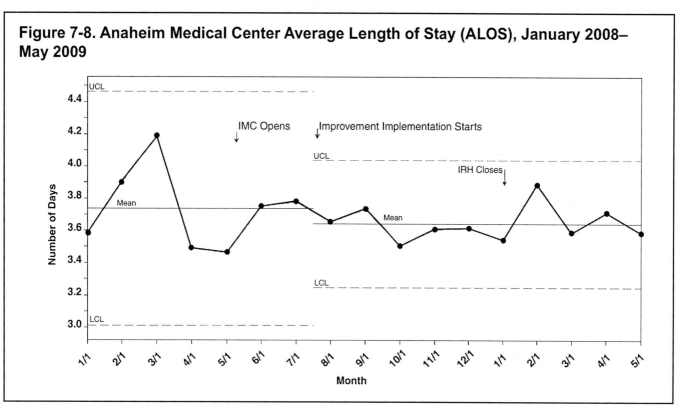

The decreasing trend in daily census before opening the Irvine Medical Center (IMC) stabilized in July–September 2008 to 135, and the census increased by 11% when the community hospital (Irvine Regional Hospital [IRH]) closed in January 2009. Mean = 3.64; upper control limit (UCL) = 4.04; lower control limit (LCL) = 3.25.

Source: *Kaiser Foundation Hospital Anaheim. Used with permission.*

Figure 7-9. Total Number of Emergency Department (ED) Visits, Anaheim Medical Center, April 2007–May 2009

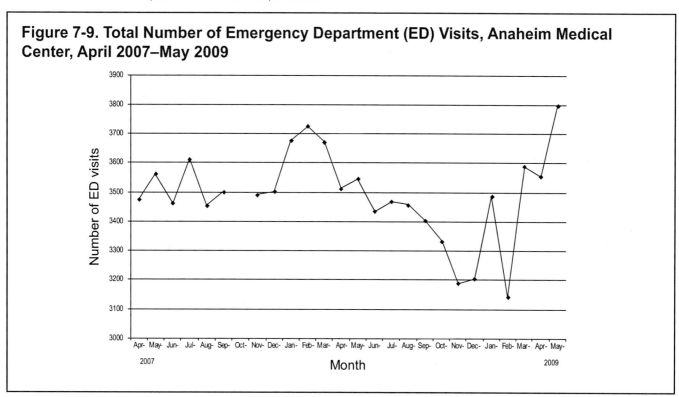

The fluctuations in the length of stay (Figure 7-8) associated with the opening of Irvine Medical Center in May 2008 and the closing of Irvine Regional Hospital in January 2009 are reflected in ED visits.

Source: *Kaiser Foundation Hospital Anaheim. Used with permission.*

Figure 7-10. Percentage of ED Patients Who Left Without Being Seen (LWBS)

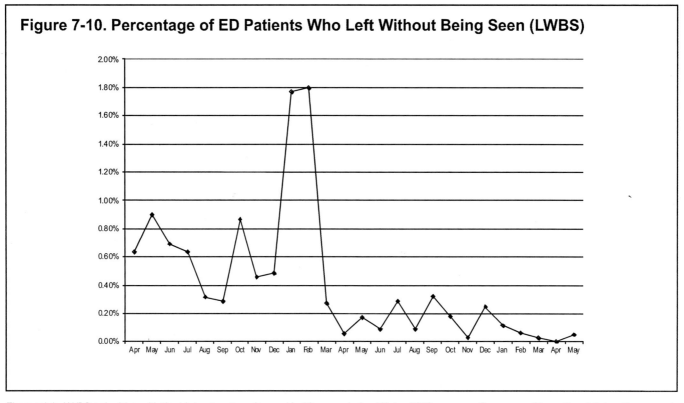

The peak in LWBS coincides with the highest system demand in 10 years during Winter 2008, a severe flu season. The national Kaiser Permanente target for LWBS is < 1%.

Source: *Kaiser Foundation Hospital Anaheim. Used with permission.*

often, projects might appear to produce useful results yet fail to produce meaningful and sustained improvement across the organization. Anaheim used system-level thinking in planning for the reduction in variation in patient flow and matching capacity to demand. Creating the driver diagram for patient flow (Figure 7-1) allowed the entire team to (1) view the organization as a system, (2) understand the interdependencies between departments and support services, and (3) create a plan to charter projects, organized by portfolios, sequenced over time that would reduce variation in the movement of patients through the system from ED through return to home. This system-level perspective also helped leaders to provide adequate resources to manage the efforts while engaging frontline staff teams in solving problems and creating better local systems of care.

Reliance on either system-level bed management or unit-level management alone could not produce better patient flow through the hospital, for both management levels needed improvements across departments, hence the creation of the cross-departmental service-level agreements. Agreement of leadership across key delivery and support functions on definitions (such as "responsive" and "timely"), prioritization of efforts, and allocation of the appropriate resources and staffing to meet patient and bed needs helped to reduce variation in staff practices and conflict between staff and departments.

When improving a system through multiple local initiatives, it is important to communicate the results and improvement frequently across the organization so that different departments can observe the effect of changes on the function of the whole system. Two key resources are essential to producing real-time information and maintaining momentum: the provision of a dedicated IA for improvement portfolios and a resource to produce data and reports so that teams can readily view progress over time.

Communication regarding the value of the work and the role of staff is essential to success. The knowledge of the roles of staff from other units, such as the ED and the ICU, in the discharge and transfer processes was enlightening for many on the team ("I didn't know that you did that"). *Knowledge of the roles and work flow is key to breaking down barriers between departments and facilitating team work.* This motivates team members, in understanding their own contributions to overall improvement, to adhere to agreed-on practices. An ICU ward clerk commented, "To have something you've implemented with your peers, and actually have it work? You never see this."

While making progress, the leadership team at Anaheim Medical Center faces challenges as it continues its patient flow improvement efforts. Given the commitment of physician time to direct patient care, the role of physician leaders has been limited to that of a champion rather than that of an active problem-solving team member. Frontline staff's resistance to change occasionally still exists, requiring active change management to facilitate change adoption. For example, the nursing staff on the team for the discharge from floor project felt uncomfortable about the change concept of asking the patient for his or her ride-home contact at the time of admission, even though nurses identified ride delay as a primary barrier to timely discharge. In the course of several team meetings, the nursing staff stated that they believed that the patient would not respond positively to this change concept. The team's co-leads then conducted an informal survey of patients on the medical/surgical unit—and found that the patients were generally willing to discuss this issue shortly after their admission. The survey was repeated twice on the same unit, with similar results. The results led the staff nurses to become more comfortable in implementing the change concept.

Sustainability plans for all of the improvement efforts include the following:

- Daily unit-level monitoring of key measures, such as length of time to transfer, discharge, or admit a patient
- Use of a bed utilization and review system that can monitor demand for staff and beds and that can match both to system-level needs on a shift-by-shift basis
- Use of an escalation report process, according to which if the receiving nurse is not available to receive the report, it is given to the buddy nurse or, in his or her absence, the charge nurse
- Monitoring of key metrics, as listed in Table 7-2, as part of a dashboard used by service-line leadership and senior operational leadership to manage system performance

The sustainability plans should help ensure that the effects of the applied processes changes do not weaken over time.

In the course of implementing the improvement efforts described in this chapter, it should be noted that they were not applied in isolation but rather concurrently with other significant changes in KP and the community at large. The opening of a second KP hospital, as described earlier, makes it difficult to determine whether the initial improvement in transfer and discharge times was a result of the patient flow efforts at Anaheim or a simple reduction in demand. However, as also noted, the improvements occurred despite the closing of the community hospital and a seasonal increase in patient acuity. Anaheim continues to apply systems thinking to better plan for the seasonal variation in acuity and continues to work on other, less predictable, factors that affect demand, such as the availability of other community resources.

In addition to spreading the sustained gains in patient flow management from Anaheim to Irvine Medical Center, KP's Southern California region is addressing the expansion since June 2009 in

the performance improvement portfolio to include reducing ED laboratory turnaround time and the length of stay of patients undergoing bowel and total joint procedures (Figure 7-1)—opportunities for improvement or levers that should enhance patient flow throughout the system.

Efforts will be initiated to understand how the system will match staffing needs to patient volumes and acuity. OR scheduling and turnaround time will be explored starting in early 2010, with the expectation that this work will improve real-time staffing management to complement the bed management system. The KP Southern California region has established a Web-based staffing program that allows for monitoring of daily staffing by unit and by shift. Key metrics available are actual, budgeted, and projected staff demand on the basis of acuity. To advance the transparency of information, KP is developing a Web-based bed board that will display units and census, with the capacity to include pending admissions and discharges. By monitoring bed availability and capacity across hospitals a health care system can assist leaders in better planning to match the staff and bed demands with actual patient numbers rather than plan for staff on the basis of seasonal or monthly numbers.

It is critical to address ongoing capacity imbalances between departments (for example, OR, ICU, and medical/surgical units). Having some departments that are understaffed and resourced while others remain overstaffed and resourced leads to an inability to respond to demand.[3] The most significant work environment stressor is increased workload.[4] All this work in patient flow management addresses patient needs for services and must be followed up by review of the roles of the entire care team. At each hospital, patient care services, the department responsible for nursing and support staff, is working with the regional patient care services department to ensure that the roles and responsibilities of the care team are revised in accordance with future work expectations. Coordinating patient care in a system where everything moves faster and more efficiently requires that an entire team, rather than a single nurse, take the responsibility of getting what is needed when it is needed for the patient.

Conclusion

Addressing whole-system improvement requires strong leadership; alignment of the leadership, staff, and physicians in a top-down focus with bottom-up improvement efforts; process redesign; systems thinking; and technological solutions—all organized around creating a culture that remains focused on meeting every patient's need for effective and efficient care.

References

1. Litvak E., et al.: Managing unnecessary variability in patient demand to reduce nursing stress and improve patient safety. *Jt Comm J Qual Patient Saf* 31:330–338, Jun. 2005.

2. Kosnik L.: Breakthrough demand-capacity strategies to improve hospital flow, safety, and satisfaction. In Hall R.W. (ed.): *Patient Flow: Reducing Delay in Healthcare Delivery. International Series in Operations Research & Management Science,* vol. 91. New York: Springer, 2006, pp. 101–122.

3. Mango P.D., Shapiro L.A.: Hospitals get serious about operations. *The McKinsey Quarterly,* May 2001, pp. 74–85.

4. French S.E., et al.: An empirical evaluation of an expanded nursing stress scale. *J Nurs Meas* 8:161–178, Fall–Winter 2000.

Chapter 8

Improving Hospitalwide Patient Flow at Northwest Community Hospital

Barbara Weintraub, R.N., M.S.N., M.P.H., A.P.N., C.E.N.; Kirk Jensen, M.D., M.B.A., F.A.C.E.P.; Karen Colby, R.N., M.S., C.N.A.A.-B.C.

From a systems standpoint, hospitals have inputs (patients coming to the hospital), throughputs (patients being treated or admitted), and outputs (patients being released). Flow is defined as the movement of these patients into, through, and out of the hospital. How efficiently this movement is accomplished determines the rate of flow through the hospital, if not throughout the entire health care system.

Many factors control the flow within a hospital. First, barriers to entry may slow or stop the flow. In the emergency department (ED), for example, the inability to get patients admitted contributes to a patient flow backlog that strains staff and creates long waits, sometimes compromising quality of care or necessitating diversions. In the ICU, transfers of patients to the floors can be delayed by the unavailability of beds, keeping patients waiting for needed ICU spaces. Patients often must be moved to less-than-ideal places because the system is not flowing smoothly, compromising the quality of patient care. Second, barriers to exit can slow or stop the flow, as well. If a patient is not discharged in an efficient and timely way, a needed and valuable space is rendered unavailable for longer than is necessary, creating backups throughout the system. Paradoxically, barriers to exit help create the barriers to entry. If inpatients cannot get out, new patients cannot get in.

As the venerable and ever-interesting Yogi Berra once said, "People don't go there anymore. It's too crowded." Although this oxymoron probably made sense only to Yogi, it is, in fact, the incentive for hospitals to work on improving patient flow and throughput. In the health care industry, patient service and patient safety are paramount. In the current economic and reimbursement climate, collecting every hard-earned dime can be tantamount to survival. The service and safety compromises, as well as the loss of income derived from hospitals going on bypass or diversion, or from patients leaving without being seen, or from prolonged inpatient stays, simply cannot be tolerated. Furthermore, although it may not be rocket science, optimizing patient flow is surprisingly analogous to it—involving getting from launch to landing quickly and safely. Throughput as a science has been around since queues, or waiting lines, were first analyzed by A.K. Erlang in 1913, in the context of telephone facilities.[1]

Industries as diverse as airlines, trucking, and fast-food drive-throughs have since made use of queuing theory, computer simulation, and demand smoothing to maximize throughput and optimize resource allocation. Despite its proven ability to better serve customers, reduce costs, and improve safety, health care has been late to jump into the science of operations management (OM) and the strategic concepts of demand-capacity matching, queuing theory, and reduction of variation to improve throughput.

Northwest Community Healthcare

Northwest Community Healthcare (NCH) is a 488-bed acute care hospital located in the northwest suburbs of Chicago. In addition to providing a full range of medically advanced inpatient and outpatient services, NCH includes the Center for Specialty Medicine, an eight-floor facility housing physician offices, medical specialty services, and advanced diagnostic technology; three ambulatory care centers; and the Day Surgery Center, The Youth Center (for adolescents with substance abuse problems), the Wellness Center (on the hospital campus), a fitness center managed on behalf of a local park district, and five medical office locations. Medical/surgical, critical care, obstetrics, cardiology, orthopedics, neurology, and gastroenterology inpatient services are provided. A supersite partnership with the local tertiary children's hospital allows NCH the opportunity to offer specialized children's services, including a pediatric emergency department and an infant special care unit.

As a large community hospital, NCH's annual volume (2008 data) consists of approximately 30,200 inpatients; 372,000 outpatients, including 74,000 ED visits; 40,000 home care visits; 3,300 newborn deliveries; and more than 18,000 inpatient and outpatient surgical cases. Medical specialties include critical care medicine, pediatrics, neonatology, emergency medicine, gastroenterology and obstetrics, surgery and surgical subspecialties of orthopedics, HEENT (head, eyes, ears, nose, and throat), a neuro-interventional program, and pancreatic surgery. NCH has more than 1,100 affiliated physicians, 4,000 employees, and 800 volunteers.

Identifying and Attempting to Address the Problem

Built in 1959, NCH has experienced rapid growth from the very beginning. Its opening on December 2, 1959, marked the culmination of a multiyear community effort that included cookie sales to raise money to build a hospital in the northwest suburbs of Chicago. Since then, the community has grown, as has the hospital's reputation, as reflected in its increasing patient population.

NCH's growth has brought about crowding, which has never fallen far off the radar and has recently become a more pressing concern. New buildings with more rooms have been added since

the hospital's inception, but crowding and suboptimal patient flow have persisted. Hospital leaders have tried a range of solutions at various times to help capacity keep pace with demand but have never reached the level of success for which they had hoped. Patient flow has been recognized as an issue at NCH in spite of acceptable results in the usual indicators of flawed flow—ED length of stay (LOS), patients leaving without being seen (LWBS), and time on diversion (*see* Table 8-1, page 131).

ED LOS was highly variable but acceptable on average. Patient placement occurred in silos, with placement processes revolving around staffing and unit processes rather than patient issues, and the focus was anywhere other than on the patient's needs and concerns. Physicians were allowed to opt their patients out of sharing double rooms and to institute their own infection control guidelines for patient placement, in spite of recommendations from the infection control department. Placement occurred via a "push process" from the sending units rather than inpatient areas "pulling" their patients from the operating room (OR), ED, or catheterization laboratory. Each inpatient unit was responsible for placing its own patients, which led to an "every person for himself or herself" mentality.

To combat these problems, the hospital has piloted multiple strategies (*see* Figure 8-1, page 131). In 1999 it contracted with a consulting group, which recommended that the hospital reconfigure the patient care delivery model by introducing the target-census concept. However, after several years, the hospital found that the concept exacerbated the patient placement problem; units were reluctant to take patients after reaching their target census. Problems with frequent full-bed alerts continued, and several units moved within the building to try to match capacity with demand by patient population. Admission nurses were introduced in 2000; their job was to initiate the voluminous paperwork that accompanies inpatient admissions to decrease the inpatient units' resistance to accepting admissions in a timely manner, reflecting the burden of admission paperwork on the inpatient nurses' workload. Unfortunately, although the inpatient nurses were grateful to be free of this paperwork (a win in the workforce satisfaction column), full-bed alerts continued—that is, there was no significant operational/throughput/capacity improvement. Subsequent innovative strategies also ultimately proved unsuccessful, including boxed lunches-to-go for discharged patients, a red–yellow–green stoplight full-bed alert plan, a new medicine/telemetry unit, and a discharge lounge for patients ready for discharge to await rides from family or friends to take them home. The problem with the discharge lounge—another care (that is, cost) site, with no income to pay for it—was that the patients using the lounge are frequently still fairly ill, confined to bed, and/or in need of medication and monitoring

Table 8-1. Emergency Department (ED) Indicators of Patient Flow, 1995 to 2008–2009*

	ED Volume	LOS - Admits	LOS - Dschgs	LOS - Total	LWBS Rate	Bypass Hrs	%Admits	EMS%
1995							19.4%	
1995-6	50,019						20.1%	
1996-77	49,557						20.1%	
1997-8	49,140						20.3%	
1998-9	51,154						21.0%	
1999-2000	53,863				0.8%		24.0%	
2000-1	57,299				0.6%	44	24.0%	
2001-2	59,550				0.6%	10.5	26.0%	24.1%
2002-3	59,383				0.4%	3	27.0%	25.9%
2003-4	61,539	4.58	2.56	3.57	0.7%	2.75	28.0%	23.3%
2004-5	65,777	4.75	5.65	5.20	0.1%	29.5	28.0%	24.4%
2005-6	69,359	4.81	2.90	3.86	0.1%	11	29.0%	27.1%
2006-7	70,886	4.69	2.89	3.79	0.1%	5.5	28.0%	27.1%
2007-8	74,674	4.78	3.06	3.92	0.1%	16.25	27.0%	27.3%
2008-9	73,000 (proj)	5.27	3.19	4.23	1.2%	0	27.0%	27.8%

*LOS, length of stay; Dschgs, discharges; LWBS, left without being seen; EMS, emergency medical services; proj, projected.

Source: *Northwest Community Hospital. Used with permission.*

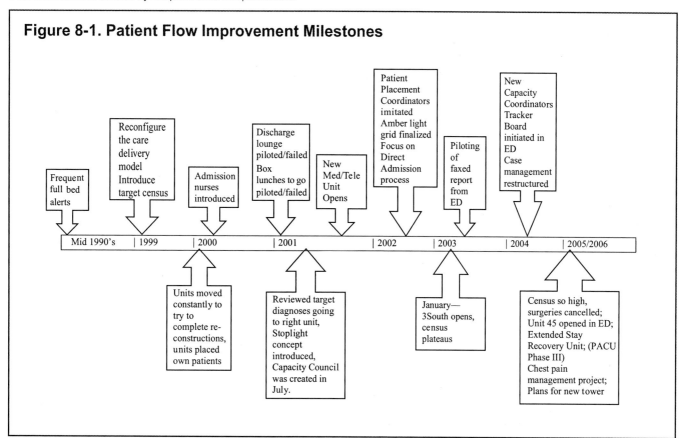

Figure 8-1. Patient Flow Improvement Milestones

The figure provides a chronology of Northwest Community Hospital's efforts to improve patient flow. Med/Tele, medicine/telemetry; ED, emergency department; PACU, postanesthesia care unit.

Source: *Northwest Community Hospital. Used with permission.*

by nursing. Nurses were therefore often reluctant to release their patients to this site, which would have necessitated another hand-off (handover). In 2001 NCH created a capacity council to bring all stakeholders to the table to cooperatively work on problem solving. The capacity council convened in times of peak census, and directors of patient care units were expected to attend. Although the meeting planners were well intentioned, the meetings revolved around brainstorming ways to increase capacity for the particular day. Unstructured as the meetings were, they generally ran between 45 and 90 minutes, and people came late and/or left early.

In 2002 NCH introduced a patient placement coordinator position, which morphed into a capacity coordinator position in 2004. These positions were created to address some of the crowding and suboptimal patient flow issues previously described and to orchestrate patient placement with an enhanced organizational overview. The nurses originally hired into the patient placement coordinator position all left the position within a year or so because of conflicts between the sending and receiving units. The inpatient (receiving) units wanted full control of which beds patients were placed in, as well as the timing of the placement (for example, waiting for the next shift to arrive to optimize staffing). The sending units, such as the ED or the postanesthesia care unit (PACU), wanted patients placed as soon as possible, in the belief that any bed was better than a holding area and that refinement in placement, such as changing roommates, could take placed later. The capacity coordinator position was created to address a number of issues, such as lack of trust or accountability on both sides, variability of processes between the capacity coordinators (who placed patients during the day) and the house supervisors (who oversaw the entire hospital and placed patients during off hours), and lack of authority to move forward with difficult decisions. However, full-bed alerts continued.

A New Start

In 2007 NCH contracted with a new physician group to staff the ED, and this group infused new energy into the patient flow improvement process. The ED medical director spent one afternoon shadowing one of the hospital capacity coordinators to see for himself the opportunities for improvement. He identified the following issues:

- The current process for ED bed request/assignment was circular (*see* Figure 8-2, page 133).
- The discharge time was not consistently articulated. Consequently, there was no incentive for either physicians or patients to plan transportation accordingly.
- There was a demand–capacity mismatch: Beds for ED admits

began to be needed by 9 A.M. (09:00), whereas beds started becoming available at 2 P.M. (14:00).

- The admission process worked as a "push," not a "pull," system.
- The authority and accountability for bed assignment was unclear (absence of ownership).
- Inpatient units were reluctant to deal with admissions during shift change (which coincides with peak admission demands).
- The system was not automated; it was entirely manual and conversational, relying on informal, narrative dialogue and negotiation rather than systematic, objective criteria.
- There were no incentives for the floors to take new patients.
- The system was reactive rather than proactive; there was little forecasting and/or planning. Inpatient staffing and processes were set up to deal with the patient population already residing on the floors, not as ready-to-serve units that routinely anticipate and plan for the ED admissions each day.
- When an admitted patient was delayed in getting to an assigned bed, the ED inconsistently communicated changes in patient status or circumstances to the target floor.

Measuring Patient Flow

Previous measures of patient flow included comparison of discharge time versus admission time, time from bed request to patient in bed, and time the patient actually left the unit versus time that this was processed in the computer. Although all these measures showed evidence of the bed crunch NCH was frequently experiencing, none revealed any obvious or easy solutions.

Various strategies were attempted to deal with individual components of these problems. The ED began faxing patient admission reports, and inpatient units were encouraged to process their discharges immediately so that the bed would show as available in the computer. However, as the story often goes, the full-bed alerts continued. A more recent measure that NCH has employed—the number of days on which NCH had full-bed alerts (*see* Figure 8-3, page 134)—provides a different view of the capacity issues. The figure provides a clear historical display of NCH's results—that despite numerous solutions tried, patient demand continued to exceed capacity.

In retrospect, some of the failings of previous efforts to improve capacity were as follows:

- The capacity council representatives were at the director level as opposed to being flow experts on the front lines.
- The capacity council lacked defined goals or purpose, and power and accountability were not allocated to the unit level.
- The capacity council did not use data to drive decisions, so improvement efforts were often driven by anecdotes, which rendered tracking of improvements impossible.

Figure 8-2. Mike's "Dancing with the Bed Czars"

1. Current process for ED bed request/assignment:

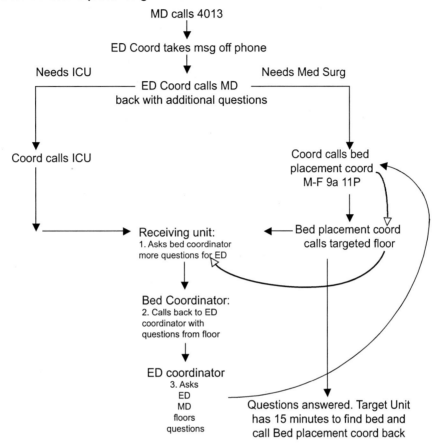

2. ***Discharge time not articulated* consistently.** Consequently there is no incentive for either physicians or patients to plan transportation accordingly.
3. ***Demand-capacity mismatch:*** Beds for ED admits begin to be needed by 9 a.m. Beds start becoming available at 2 p.m.
4. **Admission process works on a *"push"* system, not a *"pull"* system**
5. **Authority and accountability for bed assignment is unclear (absence of ownership).**
6. **Inpatient units reluctant to deal with admissions during shift change (which coincides with peak admission demands).**
7. **System is entirely unautomated, relying upon informal, narrative dialogue and negotiation, rather than systematic, objective criteria.**
8. **There are no incentives to the floors for taking new patients.**
9. **The system is reactive, rather than forecasting and planning. Inpatient staffing and processes are set up to deal with the patient population already residing on that floor, not as a ready-to-serve unit which as a matter of routine knows they will get ED admits each day, and plans for these before they are called for.**
10. **When patient is delayed in getting to assigned bed, the ED inconsistently communicates change in patient status or circumstances to target floor.**

Suggestions from Bed Placement:
1. Utilize the bed ahead system, which has fallen by the wayside.
2. Person responsible for placing patients must answer their phone.
3. When a double room is empty, leave the door closed to prevent visiting family members from seeing a potential "private" room for their family member, and requesting transfer into that room.
4. Consider ED "flow facilitator" function.

This process flow map illustrates the process for emergency department (ED) bed request/assignment before the improvement work started. MD, physician; Coord, coordinator.

Source: *Northwest Community Hospital. Used with permission.*

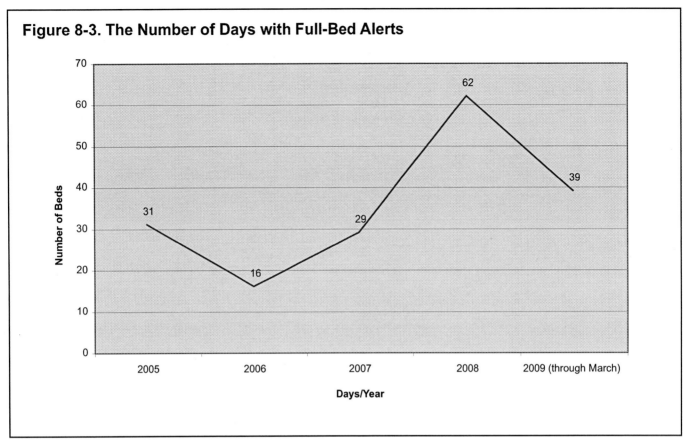

Figure 8-3. The Number of Days with Full-Bed Alerts

As shown in the figure, in spite of numerous solutions tried, patient demand continued to exceed capacity.

Source: *Northwest Community Hospital. Used with permission.*

- The length of the capacity council's meetings was often a disincentive to attend and participate. Concrete plans and solutions for the day never materialized out of the meetings, so that the value of attending was seldom appreciated, and meetings became minimally attended.

- During these meetings, individual issues, such as adequate number of pillows, were tackled, rather than organizational-level improvements, solutions, or fixes.

- The bed placement coordinators did not work 24 hours a day, 7 days a week. When they were not in the hospital, charge nurses on inpatient units were responsible for patient placement.

- When the red–yellow–green stoplight full-bed alert plan for peak census was established, all departments were involved, but the plan was not evaluated for effectiveness, departments were not held responsible for outcomes or actions, and the plan was initiated only when almost no beds were left for placement. This did not allow for proactive action or continuous learning.

If, as Albert Einstein is purported to have said, "Insanity is doing the same thing over and over again and expecting different results," then, clearly, NCH needed new strategies if it wanted new and improved outcomes or performance.

Implementation of Strategies

The One-Day Workshop. With another new patient care addition slated to open in 2010, creating yet a fifth location where patients could be placed, NCH recognized the need to develop an overarching solution that could stand the test of time. It joined the Institute for Healthcare Improvement (IHI) patient flow community[2] in 2007, with the stated goal "to create, implement, and monitor processes to provide excellent and timely care to every NCH patient at the appropriate level, in a cost-effective and quality driven manner," and patient flow was elevated to a strategic initiative in 2008.

NCH's chief nursing officer recognized that a unified, interdepartmental approach was necessary to achieve maximal patient throughput and appointed the directors of the ED and the inpatient medical units to head up the patient flow initiative. To generate interest and to launch the initiative with all stakeholders on the same page, on August 6, 2007, a kick-off full-day party/workshop, "Get a Move On: Go with the Flow," was held to introduce the initiative. A guest speaker introduced the concept of demand–capacity matching, queuing theory, and variation as it related to health care, and tables were arranged around patient flow dynamic groups (for example, OR-ICU, ICU-inpatient unit,

ED-inpatient unit), which forced each interdepartmental group to work together as a team on assignments throughout the day.

At the workshop's conclusion, the ED flow, OR, and inpatient flow teams were formed; and a patient flow steering committee (*see* Figure 8-4, below) and the peak census task force were added later. These teams set their initial purpose and goals at the workshop. Additional education was offered to the key individuals who would help lead each task force. Major strategies, such as small tests of change, building on successes, developing the ability to predict rather than react, and matching capacity to demand, were employed. The overriding theme of the day and the project in general was that patient flow is an organizational issue that affects all areas of the hospital and does not belong to only one department.

Understanding Patient Flow. To remedy a problem as large and complex as patient flow, NCH needed to understand its

foundations and the research behind the problem, so the organization undertook a review of the literature. It found that patient flow is a prime example of systems thinking—the process of understanding how the interactions of local policies and actions influence the state of adjacent systems. Systems thinking promotes approaching solutions by viewing "problems" as defects of an overall system.[3] The only way to fully understand why a problem or an element occurs and persists is to understand the part in relation to the whole.[4]

Hospital flow can be understood by using the systems model of input, throughput, and output (*see* Figure 8-5, page 136). From a systems standpoint, hospitals have inputs (patients coming to the hospital), throughputs (patients being treated or admitted), and outputs (patients being released). *Flow* is defined as the movement of patients through the system. The efficiency with which this movement is accomplished determines the rate of flow throughout the entire system. Operations management (OM), a

Figure 8-4. Patient Flow Teams

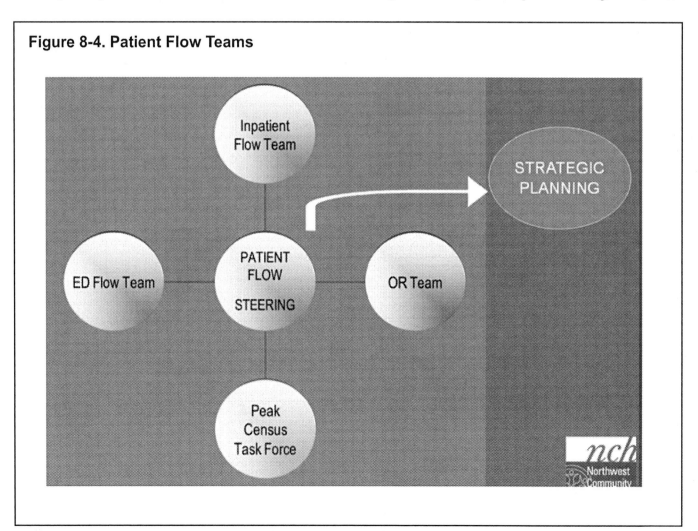

At the workshop's conclusion, the emergency department (ED) flow, OR, and inpatient flow teams were formed—and a patient flow steering committee and a peak census task force was added later.

Source: *Northwest Community Hospital. Used with permission.*

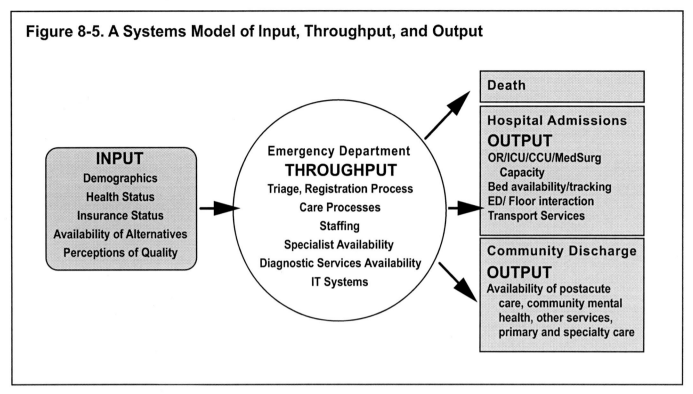

Hospital flow can be understood using the systems model of input, throughput, and output. OR, operating room; CCU, critical care unit; IT, information technology.

Source: *Northwest Community Hospital. Used with permission.*

science consisting of well-described principles that are used in many service businesses today, provides valuable tools for understanding patient flow (*see* Chapter 4). The following strategic principles are critical to OM:

- Demand capacity management
- Understanding the theory of constraints and its implications
- Queuing and queuing theory and their implications for patient flow and movement
- Variation and its impact on operations
- Real-time flow monitoring
- Forecasting and predicting of patient flow
- Demand smoothing

Operationalizing OM consists of planning and deploying service capacity to match anticipated demand. This process involves the complexities of scheduling and decreasing, adding, or adjusting capacity and must include a real-time demand capacity management system (*see* page 146). A real-time demand-capacity system (RTDC) is critical because it allows for predictions to plan for a good, bad, or average day in terms of patient flow; a bed management process; and an early-warning-and-response system. Managing capacity also includes managing the key constraints or bottlenecks. Applying the theory of constraints can be most helpful in alleviating overall bottlenecks and focusing on the critical bottlenecks. It is also necessary to understand the role that

variation plays in producing bottlenecks and to understand how to decrease that variation.

Also critical to hospitalwide patient flow is an effective administrative system, which allows key stakeholders and participants to "see flow"—making flow visible and real.

An Administrative System for Optimizing Patient Flow

An administrative system or model for optimizing patient flow includes four elements, as shown in Table 8-2 (*see* page 137).

1. Bed Management Process. The bed management process is something everyone is or should be familiar with. If you are not familiar with yours, spend an hour, a half day, or a whole day with your bed management people to get an understanding of what really goes on. The goal of bed management is to efficiently and effectively transition patients through the system. A bed management process should possess a centralized authority, convey accurate information, and have the capacity for real-time viewing.

• Possess a Centralized Authority. On the basis of its participation in the IHI patient flow community, starting in November 2007, NCH sought to improve the bed management process in several ways. First, NCH mapped the process flow (Figure 8-2)

Table 8-2. Four Elements in an Administrative System for Optimizing Patient Flow

---

1. **A bed management process**

   a. Possesses a centralized authority

   b. Conveys accurate information

   c. Has capacity for real-time viewing

2. **An early warning and response system**

3. **Long-range forecasting and planning**

   a. Theory of constraints/barriers

   b. Smoothing demand

   c. Reducing variation

4. **A real-time demand capacity system (RTDC)**

   Step 1: Predict capacity at the unit level

   Step 2: Predict demand at the unit level

   Step 3: Develop a plan for dealing with potential demand/capacity mismatches

   Step 4: Evaluate the plan: Was it successful? and lessons learned

---

Source: Northwest Community Hospital. Used with permission.

and found that it was so circular (as stated earlier) and convoluted that the ED flow team dubbed it "Mike's Dancing with the Bed Czars"—Mike being the ER medical director who mapped its choreography. There was no standard information required for requesting a bed, there were no benchmarks set for time intervals, there was no way to measure "boarding" time, and the process was highly variable and based on incomplete knowledge of bed availability. In addition, although the capacity coordinators, by job description, had the authority to place patients, they frequently had to engage in multiple negotiations to get inpatient units to take patients. In addition, there were multiple processes for placing patients:

- The process for placing patients during the capacity coordinator's hours
- The process for placing patients during the capacity coordinator's off hours
- The parallel processes that the OR and the ICU used in placing their own patients, bypassing the capacity coordinators

- Another parallel process for placing direct admissions

The ED flow team took on the bed management process as its initial project. First in line was the need to standardize the information needed to request a bed, thus reducing the variability in the system. Several renditions of a bed-request (admissions) form were tried before a final version was agreed on (*see* Figure 8-6, page 138). The major negotiations involved in fine-tuning the form involved determining which particular elements were absolutely necessary to obtain a bed. For example, inpatient units wanted to know whether the patient was oriented to person, to place, and to time. The team felt that bed placement would not differ if the patient was oriented to person and place, as opposed to place and time. The team finally agreed on "oriented × 4" or "any other ≤ × 4." As the physicians became accustomed to completing the form, the team continued fine-tuning it, eventually folding it into an admission order and initial order set (*see* Figure 8-7, page 139) and adding manual tracking times to help measure opportunities for improvement. Until then, the team had no way to measure boarding time or the time that admitted patients waited in the ED for a room. The tracking mechanism has enabled the team to report this information stat to the inpatient units and the board of directors as lost revenue opportunities, especially for the observation patients, whose official observation time starts when they reach their hospital bed.

Next, the team streamlined the process by which beds were requested, adding a fax machine to the capacity coordinator's office and faxing requests. This eliminated the triple copying of the same information as the physician called the admission line and the ED charge nurse transcribed; the ED charge nurse called the capacity coordinator, who transcribed, and then called the inpatient unit charge nurse, who then transcribed. With the initiation of the faxing component, the ED faxes the bed request to the capacity coordinator, who determines the appropriate unit and then faxes to that unit. This also eliminates the opportunity for transcription error. The team also added a text page alert to each step as a cue to check the fax machines to eliminate this as a source of error.

To centralize the patient placement authority, a revision of the capacity coordinator job description is under way. The team is also conducting small tests of change with the OR and ICU to drive all patient placements through the capacity coordinators.

• *Convey Accurate Information.* The team had multiple ways of tracking which beds the team thought were full, empty, blocked by isolation patients, and so on, but because multiple people owned pieces of the process, changes occurred in bed status in silos, making it difficult at any one time to know how many beds were available. Although an electronic bed board would

Figure 8-6. Bed Request (Admissions) Form

Admission Request

1.	From ❑ Emergency Dept# _____ ❑ Direct ❑ Transfer from _____	**Patient Sticker**

2.	**Admitting MD**		**Admit Dx:**
	Consults		

3.	**Bed type requested** ❑ Full Admit ❑ Medical ❑ Surgical ❑ Peds ❑ Psych ❑ Critical Care ❑ Observation ❑ Monitored Bed
4.	**Isolation Status** ❑ MRSA ❑ VRE ❑ PC. Diff ❑ Flu ❑ ESPL ❑ Chemo Precautions ❑ Negative Air Flow **Peds** ❑ RSV ❑ Rotavirus
5.	**Mental Status/Special Placement Needs** ❑ Normal ❑ Place Near Nursing Station ❑ Undesirable Roommate

6.	**Time Assigned Admit to RN** **Bed Status**
	 _____ Bed _____ _____ ❑ Empty Clean Ready
	                                             ❑ Empty Dirty Env Paged@ _____
	                                             ❑ Occupied Est.Empty@ _____

7.	❑ Other _____

Remember>
Do not request a bed for patients with chest pain diagnoses until receipt of the first set of enzymes!

The major negotiations involved in fine-tuning the form involved determining the particular elements that were absolutely necessary to obtain a bed.
Source: *Northwest Community Hospital. Used with permission.*

Figure 8-7. Admission Orders

1	**Bed Request**		
A	Patient Origin ❏ Emergency Dept	❏ Direct	
B	Status ❏ Inpatient: Admit to inpatient ❏ Observation: Place in observation ❏ Outpatient (To L&D, endoscopy, surgery)		
C	Admit to Dr.	Discuss with Dr.	❏ Do Not Call for routine orders
	Consult Dr.	Discuss with Dr.	❏ Do Not Call for routine orders
	Consult Dr.	Discuss with Dr.	❏ Do Not Call for routine orders
D	Preliminary Diagnoses		❏ Disposition: Critical Care
E	Allergies	❏ NKA ❏ Updated in CareLink	
F	Infectious History ❏ None ❏ MRSA ❏ Vancomycin Resistant Enterococcus(VRE) ❏ ESBL ❏ Influenza ❏ TB ❏ Rotavirus ❏ RSV ❏ Hx of C-Diff, w/active diarrhea ❏ Other___		
G	Functional Status		
	Ambulatory Status ❏ Independent ambulation ❏ Any other		
	Socialization ❏ Cooperative ❏ Combative ❏ Noisy		
	Mental Status ❏ Alert and oriented x 4 ❏ Any other (< alert & oriented x 4)		
H	Other Placement Issues ❏ Oncology (under ACTIVE Treatment) ❏ Dialysis ❏ Medication drips: ___		

2 Initial Admission Orders

❏ Telemetry monitoring   Code status ❏ Unknown ❏ _____

Routine Vital Signs per admitting unit   ❏ Neuro checks q ___ Hx ___ H

Activity ❏ Up Ad Lib   ❏ Up with assistance   ❏ Bed rest

Diet ❏ NPO ❏ Clear Liquids ❏ 1800 ADA ❏ Low Sodium ❏ Regular

IV Access ❏ Saline lock ❏ IV Fluids   Rate ___ ml/hour

O₂ Therapy

Analgesia   Medication ___ Dose ___ mg FREQq___ HPRN Pain x 2 doses

     Route ❏ IV ❏ po ❏ other___

Other Orders ___

Initiate Order Set: (Receiving RN to notify admitting physician for completion)

Cardiac	Medical	Stroke
❏ AMI	❏ DVT Accelerated Discharge	❏ Ischemic Stroke / *TIA*
❏ Chest Pain. R/O Coronary Syndrome/MI	❏ Heparin. *DVT/ PE*	❏ Ischemic Stroke/*Thrombolytic*
❏ Heart Failure	❏ Pneumonia (Adult)	❏ Other
❏ Heparin Therapy, *Angina/MI/AF*	❏ Severe Sepsis/*Septic Shock*	

Physician Signature	Physician Printed Name	Date	Time

Time: Bed Request	Time: Bed Received	Bed #	RN Assigned	Status Time ❏ Empty Clean Ready___ ❏ Empty Dirty ___ ❏ Occupied	Time: Pt leaves ED	Time: Pt arrives on floor

Northwest Community Hospital
Arlington Heights, IL 60005

1 0 4 1 5 0 R D

ADMISSION ORDERS

NCH Item# E27164   Form#003.031-209-1-ET

The admission orders form includes the original bed request form (Figure 8-6, page 138), an initial order set, and manual tracking times.
Source: *Northwest Community Hospital. Used with permission.*

alleviate this issue, the team did not yet have one so another solution was needed. The team decided to determine how many beds were available by asking each unit to bring its updated information together at the same time and place. Because all units— whether sending or receiving patients—came together at the morning bed huddle (*see* page 148), the team decided that this

was the place to begin. Because the most common complaint about previous huddle meetings was the length, the team vowed to limit the bed-huddle meeting to 20 minutes or less. To accomplish this, the team developed a spreadsheet for tracking bed availability. Each unit had its own tab for delineating its bed/patient status. The unit charge nurses felt that it would be easier to use this tool during their unit bed huddles if the form was printed out. Each unit would then write in its information and fax the form to the capacity coordinator office. The secretary in the office would enter the information into the spreadsheet tab, which then rolled up to a summary tab that provided a housewide view of bed status. Although this added a "non-value-added" step, the team felt that the process needed to be as end-user friendly as possible, even if support staff needed to work a little harder for the process to benefit frontline staff.

This spreadsheet is projected onto a screen at bed huddle each morning. At this hospitalwide huddle, each unit confirms its information, and the units then solve problems together to alleviate patient backlogs. For example, NCH now has one general postsurgical unit in operation, and most of the postoperative patients ("postops") were "scheduled" to go to them. On heavy surgical days, the demand for their beds far exceeded their capacity. What happened at these huddles, entirely without prompting, was that the unit charge nurses, aware of the fact that the unit was well over capacity (127%), would take measures to reduce the surgical unit's demand without compromising care. For example, one medical unit might volunteer to take back one of its patients who was coming in for a less complicated procedure, and pediatrics might volunteer to take a 20-year-old patient coming in for a tonsillectomy. Such actions confirm the benefits of making patient flow visible, leveling the workload, and increasing capacity and throughput.

The capacity coordinators would then leave the morning bed huddle with a hospitalwide view of predicted bed status by 2:00 P.M. (14.00) The bed-huddle spreadsheet (*see* Figure 8-8, page 141) is also available for viewing on a shared drive so that everyone from housekeeping to food services can see where NCH stands regarding patient flow.

• *Has Capacity for Real-time Viewing.* It was a challenge to provide capacity for real-time viewing in the absence of an electronic bed board. Because the bed-huddle spreadsheet is simply a spreadsheet, it would be too labor intensive to update it every hour. To get around this issue, the team implemented several solutions. First, the morning bed-huddle spreadsheet is available for everyone to view, as stated, on the hospital's shared drive. Second, when beds are particularly tight, bed huddles are repeated in the afternoon, and the bed-huddle spreadsheet is revised then. Third, to provide inpatient units a real-time view of incoming patients, the team gave each unit coordinator access to view the ED tracker board. Because the ED is responsible for 67% of the patients in hospital beds, this provides a reasonable snapshot of demand a few hours down the line. Initially, inpatient units did not find this helpful because they had no way of knowing which, if any,

of the patients in the ED were potential admits. However, the team showed the units how to use the Emergency Severity Index (ESI)[5] category on the tracker board by applying the expected number of admissions per ESI level to their own target diagnoses. With this tool in hand, inpatient units were able to determine what percentage of the patients in the ED were potential admits for them and to plan accordingly.

2. *Early Warning and Response System.* The next major component of an administrative system is an early warning and response system, which should respond efficiently and effectively to large fluctuations in demand or capacity as they are happening. To accomplish this, the team needed to be able to predict the demand for those beds and understand that the demand needs to be within the time frame of the throughput or flow goals. This is equal in effect to the need, or the queue, for those beds. McDonald's uses the official "Happy Meal Prediction Process" to have the right number of the right kind of "Happy Meals" at the right time—with the number of cars being used to make the prediction.[6] Some places that are evidently particularly savvy as about how to use queuing theory to their advantage have taken it one step further. Have you ever been to a drive-through where a worker was going from car to car, taking orders even before you got to the first window? This looks like it is done so you can give your order faster, but it works in another way as well. The worker can see how many cars in line have not yet had orders taken and can alert the inside workers to speed up (or slow down) the production process. A hospital capacity system should have the same functionality.

The stoplight plan that NCH was using—the Amber Light Policy (red–yellow–green stoplight full-bed alert plan)—as an early warning and response system was reactive rather than proactive. To develop a more proactive process, a patient flow subcommittee, the peak census task force, was established in summer 2008 to better prepare for the anticipated winter surge of patients and thus prevent subsequent delays for beds. The task force reworked the Amber Light Policy, which had no set criteria and was entirely subjective—and therefore highly variable and unreliable as either a motivator or a predictor. The new plan, the Peak Census Policy, reflected a ramping up of responses, somewhat akin to the U.S. Homeland Security Advisory System's color-coded threat level system. The team then applied conditional formatting, in which cells are formatted to turn a different color or change the font, given predefined results of embedded calculations. The team color-coded the cells in the morning bed-huddle spreadsheet, as reflected in Figure 8-8 (for example, when census/capacity met the green light level, the cells turned green, and so on) so that the appropriate peak census level would be displayed on the basis of the units' forecast of demand and capacity.

Figure 8-8. Bed-Huddle Spreadsheet

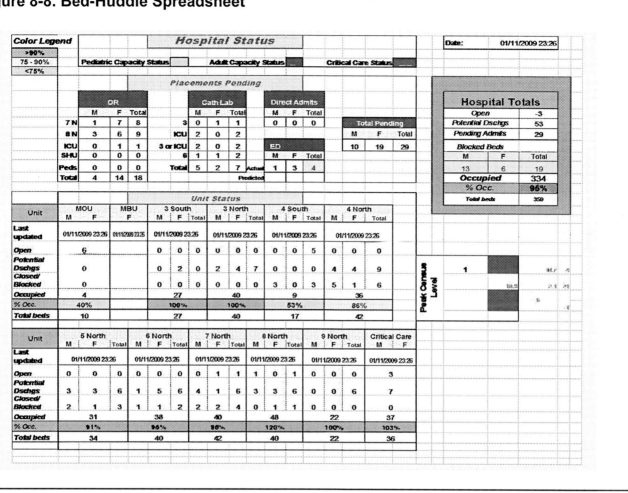

The bed-huddle spreadsheet is available for viewing on a shared drive so that everyone from housekeeping to food services can track progress on patient flow.

Source: *Northwest Community Hospital. Used with permission.*

Each clinical service as well as all the support units (for example, pharmacy, linen) was then charged with developing a departmental plan corresponding to the response level calculated on the basis of the capacity and demand. The guiding principle for writing these plans was that the majority of the work should take place at Census Alert Level 1, the lowest level. This would help prevent escalation to Levels 2 or 3, at least theoretically.

Work to refine all aspects of the early warning and response system, including the ED tracker board and the concomitant ESI education, continues. Before this coming winter's surge season, NCH plans to have each department devise a checksheet, designed from its Peak Census Policy plan, that will serve as a guide for the less-experienced charge nurses and provide a mechanism for increased accountability and feedback. A sample department-specific Peak Census Policy plan is shown in Figure 8-9 (page 143). The hospitalwide Peak Census Policy plan and a

Peak Census Policy plan checklist are provided online (http://www.jcrinc.com/MPF09/Extras).

online extras http://www.jcrinc.com/**MPF09/Extras**

3. Long-Range Forecasting and Planning. The third major component of an administrative system for optimizing patient flow, long-range forecasting and planning, can be performed on the basis of the data that a hospital typically collects. Although "long range" can mean different things to different people at different times, if the team can predict demand for a particular day, week, or holiday period, the team can allocate vacation time, time-off requests, and staffing adjustments using actual data. To do this, a hospital may need to comb through the reams of data it collects, but the effort more than pays off. By using such historical data and analyzing future projections, the team can understand and plan for variation of demand day-to-day, week-to-week, month-to-month, or year-to-year. To return to the earlier example, McDonald's uses its data to predict not only what volume to expect at any given time of day but which products are most commonly ordered in that time period. This allows them to have those products ready to go ahead of time, reducing each customer's time in the queue as well as the overall throughput time. The result? Happy customers and less hassled workers—a win–win for service and for the team.

To increase the accuracy of its bed-huddle predictions, NCH added the historical data of how many admits each inpatient unit had received from the ED, by month and by day of week, to produce the Census Summary Sheet. This allowed the units to forecast not only the number of potential admits who were in the ED but the number of potential admits who would be in the ED (*see* Figure 8-10, page 144).

• *Theory of Constraints/Barriers.* Long-range forecasting requires examining barriers to flow. Such barriers are best understood in terms of the theory of constraints, which is based on the premise that the rate of goal achievement is limited by at least one constraining process. Only by increasing flow by addressing the constraint can overall throughput be increased.[7] This can be done through the following steps:

   1. Identify the constraint/barrier (that is, the situation that prevents the organization from achieving the goal).
   2. Decide how to optimize use of the constraint (ensure that the constraint's time is not wasted doing things that it should not do).
   3. Subordinate all other processes to the above decision (align the whole system/organization to support the decision made above).
   4. Elevate the constraint (if required/possible, permanently increase capacity of the constraint; "buy more").
   5. If, as a result of these steps, the constraint has moved, return to Step 1. Don't let inertia become the constraint.

For example, in early 2009, as the team drilled down through the results culled from the Discharge Predictions Sheets used at the unit level (*see* Figure 8-11, page 145), numerous barriers were identified, as follows:

- Consulting physicians round late.
- All physicians on a case need to sign off prior to a patient's discharge.
- Intravenous (IV) pain medications are not being weaned to oral pain medications in preparation for discharge.
- Family does not pick up discharged patients until evening.

- Patients with potential need for physical therapy after discharge are not evaluated on Fridays, per physiatrist request. This delays these patients from being discharged until Tuesday.
- Delay occurs in peripherally inserted central catheter (PICC) placement.
- Delays (one- to two-hour delay from request to arrival) occur in picking up patient by ambulance companies.
- Staff R.N. occasionally delays the discharge, even after all consults have signed off on the discharge.
- Physicians covering call for their practice do not want to discharge their partners' patients.
- Discharge is postponed because the patient is scheduled to have dialysis at the hospital the next day.
- Housekeeping bed turnover is unpredictable.
- ICU beds are often unavailable because they are occupied by patients waiting to be transferred to the unit that their physician ordered, which frequently does not have room (although other floors do).

The team did a drill-down on the last two barriers, which, at least conceptually, are entirely within the control of the hospital. NCH currently has one ICU, with no designated step-down unit. As such, waits for beds in the ICU can lead to bottlenecks in the ED, OR, and cardiac catheterization laboratory. The team conducted a brief study on ICU wait time to help quantify the problem and found the following:

- Average wait times of two to four hours to transfer patients from the ICU to a medical unit
- Average wait times of three to four hours to transfer patients from the ICU to a surgical unit
- Variability between receiving units in the process of placing a patient
- Availability of beds and availability of staff for report and transport as common causes of transfer delays
- No set transfer benchmark times that were being followed

Because bed turnover was variable and unpredictable, the team sought to find the root cause(s) for this variability. On the basis of the housekeeping and the admission, discharge, and transfer (ADT) logs, the team calculated bed turnover at five days. The team then collected data on time of discharge, time housekeeping arrives, and time the bed was cleaned. To ensure consistency in data collection, the team developed a standard definition of bed turnover—the time between a discharged patient leaving the room and the bed being clean/ready for the next patient.

The team found the following:
- Average bed turnover varied each day, ranging from 120 to 180 minutes.
- Admission and discharges peak between 3 P.M. (15:00) and

Figure 8-9. Department-Specific Peak Census Plan

DEPARTMENT NAME: 2 NW Medical Pulmonary Unit
Title: **Peak Census**
Purpose: When NCH is at Peak Census (Full House) and could potentially go on bypass. This policy addresses the department of 2 NW Medical Pulmonary process to assist with patient flow during peak census periods.
Process: The following table reflects the steps in this process:

Responsible Person (s)	Procedure
Level 1 Response: Patient Care Director/Clinical Coordinator/Charge Nurse	1. Fill out bed-huddle form, update computer census every two hours. 2. Identify potential discharges. Involve unit case managers to identify patients. Work closely with physician and ancillary services to discharge patients. 3. Use tracker board to anticipate admissions from ED. 4. Cohort any patients on floor, verify with infection control if necessary following guidelines. 5. Coordinate admissions/transfers to 2 NW Medical Pulmonary with the Capacity Coordinator/Administrative Supervisor following the target census. 6. Evaluate current staffing. Place additional staff on as appropriate. 7. Evaluate unit supplies follow procedure for ordering additional supplies for increased census. 8. Evaluate patients on Central Telemetry and call for discontinue orders.
Level 2 Response: **Peak Census** Patient Care Director/Clinical Coordinator/Charge Nurse	1. Take all actions under Level I Response, above. 2. Update computer census hourly, prepare Bed Huddle Form in preparation for housewide huddle. 3. Unit huddles with staff as needed.
Level 3 Response: **Bypass** Patient Care Director/Clinical Coordinator/Charge Nurse	1. Take all actions under Level 1 and Level 2 Response, above. 2. Work closely with Capacity Coordinator/Administrative Supervisor for alternative patient care sites. 3. Cancel all meetings.

This plan specifies the processes by which 2 NW (Northwest), the medical pulmonary unit, would assist with patient flow during peak census periods. NCH, Northwest Community Hospital; ED, emergency department; CNS, clinical nurse specialist; APN, advanced practice nurse.

Source: *Northwest Community Hospital. Used with permission.*

Figure 8-10. Census Summary Sheet

Census Summary Sheet

% Occupied	
95%	
85-90%	
<85%	

Date/Time: 4/23/09 9:03 PM

UNIT	Total Beds	Discharges	Isolation	Feeder Unit Admissions M	Feeder Unit Admissions F	Available Capacity	Occupied Beds	% Occupied	Need Plan?
MOU	10	0	0	0	0	0	10	0%	No
2 South									
3 SOUTH	27	4	0	0	0	3	24	10%	No
3 NORTH	38	6	0	0	0	3	35	8%	No
4 SOUTH (PEDS)	17	1	3	0	0	9	8	5%	No
2 NW	20	3	0	0	0	1	19	3%	No
4 NORTH	19	5	5	0	0	-3	22	10%	No
5 NORTH	34	6	4	0	0	-3	37	8%	No
6 NORTH	40	4	2	0	0	-1	41	3%	No
7 NORTH	42	3	2	0	0	3	39	6%	No
8 NORTH	40	2	2	0	0	-1	41	2%	No
9 NORTH	22	2	0	0	0	1	21	6%	No
CRITICAL CARE	36	2	4	0	0	3	33	8%	No
Total Beds	345	38	22	0	0	16			No

Peak Census Level: 0

Date/Time 4/23/09 9:03 PM

UNIT	PLANS
MOU	0
2 SOUTH	
3 SOUTH	36-1 if sit test (-); 43-1 if no CP; 43-2 after EEG
3 NORTH	Beds & staffing good?
4 SOUTH (PEDS)	0
2 NW	0
4 NORTH	458-2 will probably be ready in next 2hr
5 NORTH	0
6 NORTH	cohort females
7 NORTH	am admit to different floor?; Utilize P3; Lap Chole from 5n, return to
8 NORTH	0
9 NORTH	0
CRITICAL CARE	TF & ADM
E.D.	0
Cath Lab	0
OR PACU	0
Direct Admits	0

FEEDER UNIT ADMISSIONS

	2N-W	3N	3S	4N	4S	5N	6N	7N	8N	9N	CC	SHU	ANY	MOU	Bed Requested	Bed Assn'd	Holding > 1hr
E.D. male																	
E.D. female																	
Cath Lab male																	
Cath Lab female																	
OR PACU male																	
OR PACU female																	
Direct Admits male																	
Direct Admits female																	
Total	0	0	0	0	0	0	0	0	0	0	0	0	0	0	0	0	0
Male	0	0	0	0	0	0	0	0	0	0	0	0	0	0	0	0	0
female	0	0	0	0	0	0	0	0	0	0	0	0	0	0	0	0	0

CathLab | OR_PACU | ED | InfectionCtrl | **PEAK CENSUS** | Summary | MOU | 3S | 3N | 4N | 4S | 2NW | 5N | 6N | 7N | 8N | 9N | CCU | ADMITDATA | LISTS | MasterBeds

The units use the Census Summary Sheet to forecast the number of potential admits who were and would be in the emergency department (ED). CP, chest pain; EEG, electrocardiogram; Lap Chole, laparoscopic cholecystectomy; SHU, surgical heart unit; ANY, any surgical or any medical; MOU, medical observation unit; Cath Lab, catheterization laboratory; OR PACU, operating room postanesthesia care unit.

Source: *Northwest Community Hospital. Used with permission.*

Figure 8-11. Discharge Prediction for the Next Day Form

Date_____

Rm	Name	Pt. needs prior to discharge	Confirmed	Potential	DC prior 2p	DC post 2p	Outcome, Comments and Barriers to Discharge (Check the most appropriate reason and specify)								
							MD delay	RN delay	Pt Cond	Transport delay	Test or Rx delay	Pre-Screen Or psych delay	PT OT eval	No bed @ facility	Other

Table column groups: "CM TO START THE EVENING PRIOR. UPDATE @ 8.30 AM" (Rm, Name); "CHARGE RN TO FILL-IN DURING THE 8.30AM HUDDLES." (Pt. needs prior to discharge, Confirmed, Potential, DC prior 2p, DC post 2p); "AT CHANGE OF SHIFT, FILL OUT THE CAUSE IF THE PATIENT DOES NOT LEAVE AS PREDICTED" (Outcome, Comments and Barriers to Discharge)

The case manager completes this form, in which he or she predicts which patients will be ready to leave the next day, before leaving for the day. The form is then rereviewed and updated by the evening and night charge nurses, and the day charge nurse uses it the next day for the unit's morning bed huddle. R.N., registered nurse; Rm, room; Pt., patient; DC, discharge; 2p, 2 P.M. (14:00); Cond, condition; Rx, treatment; psych, psychiatry; PT, physical therapy; OT, occupational therapy.

Source: *Northwest Community Hospital. Used with permission.*

6 P.M. (18:00), which means increased demand for housekeeping services at that time.

- Housekeepers are assigned to more than one floor during the afternoon shift, identified as the time of highest demand for housekeeping room cleans.
- Assigned housekeeper does not make regular rounds to check for patient discharges.
- Housekeeping supervisor may pull the housekeeper from one floor to another to respond to a stat clean. Because regular rounds are not made, all rooms needing cleaning on afternoons are marked "stat."
- The unit secretary communicates discharge time to the housekeeper via an ADT log. If there is a delay in transcribing the discharge time and room number to the log, the housekeeper is not aware of the dirty bed, and the room does not get cleaned.
- Each housekeeper has a cleaning cart that he or she is responsible for maintaining. There is also a stat cart. Housekeepers are reluctant to use "their" cart when called to do a stat on another floor, so they wait for the elevator to take them to the floor the stat cart is on, wait again to go down to the floor the clean is on, then wait again to return the cart when they are done. (You must admire the diligence with which the housekeepers maintain their supplies!)

Since May 2009, NCH has implemented the following strategies, currently in process, to address these issues:

1. Standardize the process for notification of stat cleans. Use text paging for stat cleans and vancomycin-resistant enterococcus (VRE)/airborne precaution room cleans during the afternoon shift.

2. Housekeepers will include the time of patient discharge in their log.

3. For all stat cleans, the housekeeper will notify the ED charge nurse via pager when the bed is clean.

4. In an effort to improve communication, the discharge escort will enter the time of discharge on the discharge slip (*see* Figure 8-12, page 146) and hand it to the unit secretary.

5. The inpatient flow committee co-chairs will meet with the housekeeping supervisor to discuss hourly floor rounds by the designated housekeeper to check for discharges.

To further reduce bed turnover delays, a housekeeping task force was established in Spring 2009 to identify additional process improvements. The task force's July 2009 drill-down study, Reducing Bed Turnover Delays (http://www.jcrinc.com/MPF09/extras), features additional findings and recommendations. The task force also created a protocol, Housekeeping

Figure 8-12. Patient Discharge Passport

PATIENT DISCHARGE PASSPORT

Patient ID label

DC Time_____

Transporter please place in basket
@ the front station

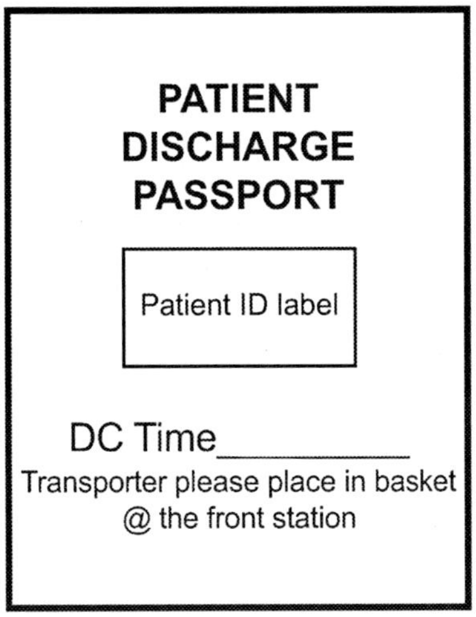

The discharge escort enters the time of discharge on this form and hands it to the unit secretary. ID, identification; DC, discharge.

Source: *Northwest Community Hospital. Used with permission.*

Process Flow for PM Shift (http://www.jcrinc.com/MPF09/ extras), to delineate housekeeping responsibilities and procedures.

Online extras http://www.jcrinc.com/MPF09/Extras

• *Smoothing Demand.* Smoothing demand is another concept that is important in improving patient flow. Intrinsic to optimization of health care is the understanding that patients with variable conditions requiring variable resources present at variable times to receive care from providers with variable levels of expertise and experience. This random variability cannot be eliminated, but if its impact is lessened and nonrandom variability is controlled, patient flow can be improved.[8] Nonrandom variability is often driven by individual priorities. For example, surgical schedules may be heavy on Wednesdays but light on Fridays, reflecting surgeons' preferences rather than actual demand. Nonrandom variability should not be managed; it should be eliminated.[2] Surgical schedules are typically a major source of nonrandom variation because of physician preference for block scheduling.

Another source of nonrandom variation in the OR is nonadherence to start times. In late 2008, the OR team began its first small test of change by enlisting one of the general surgeons to kick off the flow initiative by enforcing the 7:30 A.M. (07:30) start time in one OR. This exercise was especially interesting because the definition of *start time* varied among surgeons, preop-

erative-area nurses, anesthesiologists, and perioperative nurses. Although this process met with a fair amount of resistance at the outset, the nurses and surgeons in the designated 7:30 A.M. (07:30) start room were delighted because they found they started when they thought they would, ended when they thought they would, and required "staying over," or overtime, less frequently. This was a win–win for all involved. This concept was soon carried over to a second OR, a second day, and a second surgeon.

The OR staff became so engaged in the patient flow improvement process that an outside consultant was engaged to identify further opportunities to maximize use of costly OR resources, minimize overtime, minimize delays in scheduled cases, and smooth utilization to avoid over and underutilization of OR staff and rooms.

• *Reducing Variation.* Reducing variation is the last concept for the long-range forecasting and planning component of the administrative system for optimizing patient flow. Some of the bigger wins in reducing variation have been discussed elsewhere, including standardizing the admission data set, the ED bed request process, and the redesign of the capacity coordinator role, as well as many of the OR initiatives.

4. Real-time Demand Capacity (RTDC). The fourth major component of an administrative system is the RTDC system— basically, the patient flow equivalent of a global positioning system (GPS). RTDC tells you not only where you are (capacity) but where you're going (demand). This patient flow GPS must have certain characteristics and, most importantly, must actually work in the real world—which is not easy to accomplish.

In implementing RTDC at NCH, because of the enormity of the project, NCH chose the IHI framework,[2] which consists of the following four steps: (1) Predict capacity at the unit level; (2) predict demand at the unit level; (3) develop a plan for dealing with potential mismatches at the unit level (the plan may have system components as well); and (4) evaluate the plan.

• *Step 1. Predict Capacity at the Unit Level.* The patient flow steering committee arrived at a consistent definition of *capacity*— discharges plus available beds at the beginning of the designated time interval. The committee chose the interval of 8:30 A.M. (08:30; the time of the unit bed huddles) to 2:00 P.M. (14:00). Using flow RTDC[2] and the lessons learned in the IHI flow community, the committee performed a series of activities to design a system to accomplish this step:

■ Identify a consistent definition of discharge: The patient physically left the patient room and will not return to that bed.

■ Develop a method to predict the number of discharges from a unit within a specific time interval (for example, 8:30 A.M. to 2 P.M. [08:30–14:00]). The reliability of the prediction of discharges should be evaluated at the end of the time interval.

■ Develop a process (who, what, where, when, how) on the units to gather the information needed (for example, potential discharges, discharges with written orders).

■ Predict the current reality. Try to avoid taking on specific improvement projects until predictions are reliable.

■ Improve the prediction formula through repeated testing and by learning from inaccurate predictions. Collect information for four to five days before changing the formula. Do not deliberately underestimate the number of discharges because doing so will affect the integrity of the subsequent plan.

To develop a process to predict capacity, in November 2007 the patient flow steering committee decided that the initial test of change to predict capacity would start with 6 North, an inpatient medicine unit. This unit was ideal for the following reasons:

■ The culture of this unit was one of change and innovation. For example, the unit had participated in previous patient care improvement projects and was open to changes in work flow processes.

■ The unit was particularly interested in having more predictability and control over its patient flow.

■ The unit reported to one of the co-chairs of the patient flow steering committee.

The initial test of change chosen was to formalize the process for predicting discharges. The patient flow steering committee began by enlisting the case managers, who are unit based. A case manager's role was to list those patients whom he or she felt were potential discharges for the next day. The next morning, the bed huddle on the unit began with the case manager, the bedside nurses, and the unit manager conducting a collaborative review of this list. After reviewing the predictions from the previous day, they updated the list of the patients whom they felt were definite or probable discharges that day. The goal was to create a list with an accuracy rate of 80%. The model, methods, and calculations were refined and rerefined to improve the prediction formula through repeated testing and learning from inaccurate predictions until they refined their process every day until each day's prediction reached the goal of an accuracy rate of 80% (Figure 8-11). At that point, the prediction analysis was rolled out to the other two medicine units managed by the same director.

As the case manager, the bedside nurses, and the unit manager on 6 North were refining their predictions, they noticed an unexpected but consistent effect of their efforts. As they worked to better predict discharges, they opened up beds earlier in the day. Because they had the most open beds when the ED began admit-

ting, they started receiving a disproportionate number of admissions from the ED. This led to the first "A-ha" moment, and, accordingly, the team rolled out future efforts on all the medicine units simultaneously to avoid the "penalized for success" paradox.

Members of the inpatient flow team had several other "A-ha" moments as the unit worked on perfecting its predictions. Unit charge nurses were initially reluctant to make the determination that a patient was ready for discharge if there was no discharge order written. In response, the team tried reinforcing the concepts that (1) these were only predictions—so that incorrect predictions were not a bad thing, and that (2) the charge nurses, as experienced caregivers, were intimately aware of when patients had reached the goals necessary to achieve discharge. Yet the fear of making an incorrect prediction proved to be a very powerful cultural barrier to overcome. To avoid being wrong, nurses either listed no one or everyone as a possible discharge, depending on how they defined *possible*. The team made several alterations in some of the tools to assist the nurses past this barrier, as follows:

■ The team added space on the unit bed huddle spreadsheet so that nurses could list "definite (orders written) discharges" versus "predicted (ready to go but no order written) discharges." This allowed the nurses to use their judgment without going out on a limb and saying a patient could go before the physician had written the order.

■ The team offered several educational sessions at monthly clinical coordinator meetings on how "being wrong" in predictions helped us uncover barriers, which the team could then work to resolve.

■ The team refined the unit discharge prediction tool (Figure 8-11) to help clarify the interrelatedness of prediction failure and barrier identification.

• *Step 2. Predict Demand at the Unit Level.* While each unit is able to independently determine its capacity, collaboration with the sending units is necessary to properly determine demand. The team defined demand—the number of admissions (that is, patients needing a bed on an inpatient unit) from the various streams (for example, ED, direct admissions, PACUs, ICU transfers) into a unit during a specific time interval (for example, 8:30 A.M. [08:30] to 2 P.M. [14:00]).

Step 2 consisted of the following activities, which the team carried out as part of NCH's membership in the IHI flow community:

■ Develop a process to gather the information needed for predicting demand (consider known admissions first).

■ Using the information gathered, predict the number of admissions during the "time interval."

■ Gather historical data on admissions to refine the prediction.

NCH offers the following tips and key considerations:

■ Consider known admissions first—that is, patients already in the ED or PACU, patients on the surgery schedule, and patients scheduled for a direct admit or an internal transfer.

■ Collecting months of historical data on admissions is usually not helpful; the previous few weeks is usually sufficient.

■ Ensure that predicted admissions reflect those patients who need to be placed in an inpatient bed in a specific time interval to meet agreed-on throughput goals. For example, if a hospital's ED door-to-floor goal is four hours, a patient who will be admitted who arrives in the ED at 8 A.M. (08:00) will need to be included in the predicted admissions before 2 P.M. (14:00), while one arriving at 11 A.M. (11:00) would not.

■ Improve the formula for predicting admissions through repeated testing and learning after studying the reasons that the prediction failed.

■ Divide all the admissions among the multiple units in the medical service by some articulated method (for example, divide equally, divide on the basis of the historical number of admissions).

To achieve the goal of bringing all the information together to a "centralized authority," in February 2008 NCH instituted hospitalwide unit bed huddles. Additional aspects of the morning bed huddles not already outlined are as follows:

■ Bed huddles are held Monday through Friday, 9:30 A.M. (09:30); they are usually not held on weekends or holidays, although the supervisor can always call for one if needed, such as on a weekend day when patients are boarded in the ED or if the ICU is full.

■ Representatives from each inpatient unit, the ED, the OR, the catheterization laboratory, infection control, housekeeping, and case management attend.

■ The decision for peak census is made on the basis of demand (incoming) and capacity (empty beds and potential discharges) reported at the huddle.

• Step 3. Develop a Plan for Dealing with Potential Mismatches at the Unit Level. After processes are developed to predict demand as well as capacity, they should be compared. If the prediction of demand exceeds the prediction of capacity, a plan for matching them is needed. A plan includes articulation of the specific adjustments (for example, arranging a ride for a patient from the hospital to home) required either by the unit or the hospital to match predicted capacity to predicted demand. In this step, the focus should be on developing a plan and testing adjustments when demand exceeds capacity. If the prediction of admissions and the prediction of capacity are matched or predicted capacity is greater than the prediction of admissions, no plan is needed.

Step 3 consisted of the following activities[2]:

■ Document and test actions that can be made at the unit level if a plan is needed (consider unit bed huddles).

■ Document and test actions that can be made at the system unit level if a plan is needed.

■ Develop a process to share the plan (consider revising the hospital bed meeting).

NCH offers the following tips and key considerations:

■ Unit-level adjustments in the plan will require personal involvement from frontline staff. Adjustments will be specific to a given patient (for example, needs a laboratory test, physical therapy, a ride, a prescription written). Frontline staff will know the barriers and how to make the adjustments work.

■ If unit adjustments are insufficient to develop a successful plan, system-level adjustments (for example, hospitalists expediting the discharge of patients from certain units, director of radiology moving up the priority of an x-ray for a particular patient, opening a flex unit) need to be considered.

■ Plans should be unique on the basis of the current circumstances rather than from a list of unproven and generic possible solutions.

■ The focus of the formal all-hospital bed meeting should be on units that need plans and whether system-level adjustments are necessary. For example, suppose critical care is full to capacity (36 beds). The ED is holding 3 patients who need critical care beds, and the cardiac catheterization laboratory has several patients who may also need a critical care bed. In summary, critical care's capacity at this point is 0, it has no empty beds, but its demand is 3 or more, depending on the patients in the catheterization laboratory. Because the demand exceeds capacity, it needs a plan. To make room, it needs to transfer patients to other units. There are patients on the cardiac step-down unit who could be discharged if they could get their stress tests early in the day, rather than late. Thus, creating capacity in critical care requires a collaborative effort by critical care, the step-down unit, and cardiac diagnostics. This is a systems-level adjustment—required interventions go beyond what critical care could accomplish independently.

■ The unit-level plan should be in the form of a written document, both for clarity and to analyze the plans for success or failure.

To assist each unit in creating specific plans, the plan that each unit develops in response to their predicted demand capacity situation is transcribed to the hospital bed-huddle spreadsheet (Figure 8-10). The column "Need plan?" is conditionally formatted to compare the two calculations—predicted demand and predicted capacity—and to display "Yes" or "No" on the basis of that calculation. The team added the "Need Plan?" column recently because the concept was unclear to many staff.

Housewide bed huddles have been in place for more than 18 months now, with great success, reflecting the required collaboration. Every day the formal all-hospital bed meeting team gathers and reviews the flow from all departments. To elevate the level of awareness for the patient flow project, an organizationwide newsletter was developed that reports current patient flow processes and successes. The newsletter, *Get a Move On, Go with the Flow* (named after the initial day-long presentation) was e-mailed to all hospital employees to emphasize the concept of patient flow as an organizationwide initiative.

• *Step 4. Evaluate the Plan for Dealing with Potential Unit-Level Mismatches.* At the end of the specified time interval, the plan's success needs to be evaluated. Develop a process (who, what, where, when) to evaluate the plan. The evaluation could be done at an afternoon bed meeting or could be assigned as a role to a person such as the patient placement coordinator. If both the demand and capacity elements of the plan are successful, the plan is thought to have worked. Otherwise, the plan "failed."

The important next and necessary step is the reflection and learning that comes as a result of asking "why" if the plan failed. This includes situations where the unit team did not formulate a plan but has since learned that it should have; deciding "we did not need a plan" is actually a plan. If the plan did not work, the team should study both the adjustments included in the plan and the initial predictions of discharges and admissions as potential sources for improving the plan. If a plan was developed and it worked, cataloging the unit- and system-level adjustments that were part of the plan for future use in similar circumstances can be most helpful for learning and system improvement. The team also has the opportunity to determine whether there are system changes that could be tested and implemented to eliminate the need for adjustments that are routinely made at the unit or system level (for example, if there is always a need to expedite an MRI, create specified time slots early in the day for a certain number of MRIs).

Results

Soon after beginning the patient flow project, NCH discovered a lack of data collected for consistent measures. There were no processes in place to collect data, nor any consistent definitions by which the team could even define data points. In spite of these barriers, using the bed request and initial orders set (Figure 8-7), NCH has been able to collect data for the measures shown in Table 8-3 (*see* page 150).

As shown in Table 8-3, between 2005 and 2009, the ED census increased by almost 12% from 56,157 to an estimated 60,853, while the overall average LOS decreased by 3.2%, from 3.86 hours to 3.73 hours. For the same period, the average admissions LOS (from time of triage to time the patient leaves the department) increased by only 2.1%, from 4.81 hours to 4.91 hours. The average length of time from a bed request to the patient's placement in the inpatient unit increased from 122.1 minutes to 137.4 minutes, a 12.5% increase, but the percentage of patients for that same interval also increased for the same period, from 57.6% to 63.8%. This translated to a greater percentage of patients making to their destination within our goal time (90 minutes), but wider variation in times during periods of high census. Improved performance is also reflected in decreased bed turnover times—from 120 to 160 minutes in February 2009, when NCH began to put new patient flow processes in place, to 105 minutes in June 2009. Our next goal is reduce bed turnover times to 90 minutes and eventually reach the benchmark goal of 55 minutes.

Discussion

In many hospitals, a rallying cry of "Everyone out by 10 A.M.!" drives the patient discharge system. The short- and long-term goal of the "10 A.M." (10:00) call effort is to open up inpatient bed capacity. As described in this chapter, delays, disruptions, and barriers slow or stop the flow of patients through the hospital. As they currently operate, most hospital flow systems are push systems—patients are pushed through as staff try to coordinate a complex series of events on a schedule that is impossible to meet. NCH has learned that patient flow, as a property of the entire acute care system, can only be truly optimized at the system level—it cannot be optimized at the individual microsystem or unit level. This systemwide viewpoint presented a challenge, given that many units and departments attempt to optimize patient flow in their individual units and patient care areas, which can inversely affect other areas of the patent flow spectrum. This is not a case of people behaving badly on the unit level. Simply optimizing patient flow in their respective units makes sense if one is not plugged into (or aware of) the big picture—the system as a whole. The bed control/patient flow coordinators could not and cannot accomplish consistent optimization of demand and capacity on a shift-by-shift and day-by-day basis on their own.

Taking a hospitalwide approach has enabled NCH to improve the management of patient flow, increase bed capacity, engage staff, and improve service. NCH will continue to focus on strategies and tools required to improve flow across the acute health care spectrum, including the administrative system, with its emphasis on RTDC.

Table 8-3. Average Time for Bed Requests to Patient in Bed and < 90-minute Time from Bed Requested to Patient in Bed, 2004–2009*

Census			
2004 - 2005	56157		
2005 - 2006	59311		
2006 - 2007	60256		
2007 - 2008	62757		
2008 - 2009	60853	est	11.8%

Avg time - Bed Request - Patient in Bed		
2006	122.1	
2006 - 2007	120.5	
2007 - 2008	125.3	
2008 - 2009	137.4	12.5%

% < 90 min - Time from Bed Requested - Patient in Bed		
2004 - 2005	57.56%	
2005 - 2006	67.76%	
2006 - 2007	69.86%	
2007 - 2008	69.75%	
2008 - 2009	63.76%	9.1%

ALOS - Average Length of Stay	Admit	D/C	Total		
2005 - 2006	4.81	2.90	3.86		
2006 - 2007	4.69	2.89	3.79	Increase 2009 over 2004	
2007 - 2008	4.78	3.06	3.92	Admit	Total
2008 - 2009	4.91	3.11	3.73	2.1%	-3.2%

*For 2004–2005, 2006–2007, and 2007–2008, data are shown for October to September; for 2008–2009, data are shown for October 2008 to June 2009.

Source: Northwest Community Hospital. D/C, discharge. Used with permission.

Flow is a complex technical problem that cannot be solved by any one hospital department acting as an independent agent. Optimal solutions have required high levels of both cooperation and integration. The solution cannot be installed or be force-fed into compliant units. Principles, models, tactics, and strategies—including matching capacity to demand, reducing variation, queuing, the theory of constraints, system redesign, forecasting, and shaping demand—can and should be used. Success requires effective diagnosis of the problems, application of the relevant strategies and tactics, and effective testing of the changes using multiple plan–do–study–act cycles.

The initial time and effort involved in educating and engaging NCH staff was significant. Moving from a reactive, crisis-driven approach to a proactive and predictive model was not an easy feat. Education, rapid-cycle testing, and a healthy sense of experimentation, exploration, prototyping, and improvement were essential. The early development and engagement of educated, committed, and enthusiastic champions—at both the unit and hospitalwide levels—was critical to NCH's success. Continuous reinforcement and optimization of the process and procedure and training new people in this approach to patient flow, all the while monitoring key process and outcome measures, is still under way. Making the process, measures, and outcomes transparent to key stakeholders has proven to be a necessary component of NCH's revised approach to patient flow. Deterioration of a good but relatively new process over time is always a threat and will require vigilance and commitment.

The business case is strong—the cost of poor patient flow includes ED diversions, staff overtime, lost capacity, and the costs of rework and medical errors. The return on investment can be high for each incremental improvement in bed turns and bed capacity. Facing unmet demand for services and improving the impediments to good patient flow should make for a healthy contribution to NCH's bottom line. NCH's improvement and change management efforts involved an investment of management and performance improvement time, but no new staff were added, and no significant capital outlays were required.

Recommendations

Our recommendation for others who would undertake this work would be to understand the key strategies in improving patient flow management:

- Develop a robust and reliable administrative system
- Undertake RTDC management
- Develop interventions based on understanding the causes of your delays, identifying and capturing ways to optimize flow and increase capacity
- Understand the concept of the flow patient streams through the hospital
- Focus on key interventions that reduce or eliminate critical constraints
- Eliminate and smooth variation

Conclusion

This has been a fascinating, challenging, and exciting adventure for NCH, and it has led to improvements in patient flow and capacity that have benefited both patients *and* staff.

Aristotle, perhaps the first systems engineer, put it this way: "We are what we repeatedly do. Excellence is not an act but a habit."

References

1. Singh V.: *The Collected Works of Vikas Singh: Use of Queuing Models in Health Care.* http://works.bepress.com/vikas_singh/4 (accessed Aug. 26, 2009).
2. Institute for Healthcare Improvement (IHI): *Optimizing Patient Flow: Moving Patients Smoothly Through Acute Care Settings.* IHI Innovation Series white paper. Boston: IHI, 2003 (available on http://www.IHI.org; accessed Aug. 26, 2009).
3. O'Connor J., McDermott I.: *The Art of Systems Thinking: Essential Skills for Creativity and Problem-Solving.* San Francisco: Thorsons Publishing, 1997.
4. Capra F.: (1996) *The Web of Life: A New Scientific Understanding of Living Systems.* New York: Anchor Books, 1996.
5. Agency for Healthcare Research and Quality (AHRQ): *Emergency Severity Index, Version 4: Implementation Handbook.* http://www.ahrq.gov/research/esi/esi1.htm (accessed Aug. 26, 2009).
6. Shropshire C.: Fast-food assistant "Hyperactive Bob" example of robots' growing role. *Pittsburgh Post-Gazette,* Jun.16, 2006. http://www.post-gazette.com/pg/06167/698696-96.stm#ixzz0LoA30n73Pittsburgh Post-Gazette (accessed Aug. 26, 2009).
7. Cox J., Goldratt E.M.: *The Goal: A Process of Ongoing Improvement.* Croton-on-Hudson, NY: North River Press, 1986.
8. Litvak E: Optimizing patient flow by managing its variability. In *From Front Office to Front Line: Essential Issues for Health Care Leaders.* Oakbrook Terrace, IL: Joint Commission Resources, 2005, pp. 91–111.

Index

Letters following page numbers indicate figures *(f)*, tables *(t)* and sidebars *(s)*.

W